DATE DUE

Choreographing
ASIAN AMERICA

Choreographing
ASIAN AMERICA

Yutian Wong

WESLEYAN UNIVERSITY PRESS
Middletown, Connecticut

Published by Wesleyan University Press, Middletown, CT 06459
www.wesleyan.edu/wespress

Printed in U.S.A.

5 4 3 2 1

Portions of chapter 1 and the epilogue originally appeared in "Towards a
New Asian American Dance Theory," *Discourses in Dance* 1.1 (2002):
69–89.

Library of Congress Cataloging-in-Publication Data
Wong, Yutian.
Choreographing Asian America / Yutian Wong.
   p. cm.
Includes bibliographical references and index.
ISBN 978-0-8195-6703-1 (pbk. : alk. paper)
ISBN 978-0-8195-6702-4 (cloth)
1. Dance—Anthropological aspects—United States. 2. Choreography—
United States. 3. Asian Americans—Ethnic identity. 4. Asian Americans—
Cultural assimilation. 5. Asian Americans and mass media. I. Title.
GV1588.6.w66 2010
792.80895073—dc22   2009036033

Wesleyan University Press is a member of the GreenPress Initiative.
The paper used in this book meets their minimum requirement for
recycled paper.

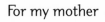
For my mother

CONTENTS

ACKNOWLEDGMENTS

This book could not have materialized without the support and guidance of family, friends, and colleagues. First I would like to express my gratitude to my dissertation advisors, Marta Savigliano and Susan L. Foster, for believing that my half-formed ideas could become a field of study and to Suzanna Tamminen for seeing the project to its end. Time to think, and write, was made possible by an Andrew W. Mellon Postdoctoral Fellowship at Bryn Mawr College, an Illinois Program for Research in the Humanities Faculty Fellowship, and a Research Board Grant from the University of Illinois, Urbana-Champaign.

Over the years numerous people have provided invaluable feedback as the work emerged in both its written, spoken, and performed iterations. I thank Priya Srinivasan, Lucy Mae San Pablo Burns, San San Kwan, Esther Kim Lee, Sean Metzger, Dan Bacalzo, Karen Shimakawa, Josephine Lee, and Anthea Kraut for years of listening. Their insights are reflected on the pages of this book. I want to thank the artists who shared their work with me including Hung Nguyen, Hiep Nguyen, Ham Tran, Uyen Huynh, Jayvee Hiep Mai, Sue Li-Jue, Maura Nguyen Donohue, and Erin O'Brien. The Asian American Studies Program at the University of Illinois, Urbana-Champaign provided an intellectual home for this work. Thank you to Kent Ono, Augusto Espiritu, Martin Manalansan, Lisa Cacho, David Coyoca, Junaid Rana, Moon-Kie Jung, Yoon Pak, Lisa Nakamura, Mary Ellerbe, Pia Sengsavanh, and Viveka Kudaligama. A thank you to the School of Music and Dance at San Francisco State University for welcoming me into a spirited community of faculty and students.

Jens Richard Giersdorf, Denise Uyehara, Fiona I.B. Ngô, Mimi Nguyen, Soo Ah Kwon, Christopher Lee, Michael Masatsugu, and Brian Locke have provided love, food, and friendship to survive the ups and downs of academic life. From my family I have inherited a number of things that have manifested in this work for better or worse. From my *gonggong* and *popo* I have inherited a love of a good anecdote told with a sense of drama, from my *mama* a love of dancing, and from my *baba* a love of reading. That I would one day write an ethnography on Asian American dance theater was perhaps inevitable. My brother Yu-Tung has provided steadfast support, and my sister Adrienne has provided the personalized cheerleading that only an astrological twin can channel.

Most of all I thank my sweetheart Bruce and my son Blake, whose very first words included "sing the book."

Introduction

Can you name an Asian American choreographer? I asked this question years ago when I choreographed my first dance. No one could give me an answer. There I was in the studio, sweating and taking inventory of each newly discovered ache in my back, trying to make sense of my double life performing as Miss Moon Festival contestant number ten and as an aspiring, angst-ridden Asian American choreographer. Both performances claimed to represent the voice of an Asian American community, yet each followed different aesthetic and political agendas.

Two performances by Alvin Ailey American Dance Theater and Dance Theatre of Harlem inspired my first forays in choreography. Alvin Ailey American Dance Theater's production of Jawole Willa Jo Zollar's *Shelter* and Dance Theatre of Harlem's *Firebird* staged black bodies that had nothing to do with the racial stereotypes perpetuated by mainstream media. This was self-representational work that married to-die-for six o'clock extensions with social commentary—I thought I was in heaven. More importantly, the sheer number of black bodies on stage heightened the whiteness of the dance studios I had spent my life in. If dancing assumes looking at the body, these choreographers shifted my looking. These works prompted me to question how I looked at dancing bodies, how race functions in the dance studio, and, finally, why I could not name a single Asian American choreographer.

Choreographing Asian America examines the relationship between Asian America and American dance history and the attendant disciplinary, political, methodological, and aesthetic concerns. With a focus on Club O' Noodles (CON), the first Vietnamese American performance ensemble established in the United States, this study makes the work of a Vietnamese American performance collective central to an investigation of Asian American dance. Founded in 1993 by Hung Nguyen and Tram Le, this Los Angeles–based company was the first Vietnamese American performance ensemble dedicated to articulating a bicultural perspective of living as Vietnamese refugees and immigrants in the United States.

Guided by Nobuko Miyamoto, a pioneer of the Asian American theater scene in the 1960s, Club O' Noodles's performance aesthetic in the mid- to late 1990s drew upon modern and postmodern dance techniques, song, poetry, and spoken dialogue to craft performances that called attention to the Vietnamese American experience in the United States. The company sought to integrate Vietnamese American identity into the narrative of American national identity that found the term "Vietnamese American" irreconcilable within American narratives of the Vietnam War, and to create an alternative site for Vietnamese American artists to stage multidisciplinary dancetheater productions.[1] I use the term "dancetheater," derived from the German *tanztheater*, to account for the multidisciplinary and theatrical elements of Club O' Noodles's work. Dancetheater, broadly defined, combines choreographed movement, spoken text, singing, and other media (projections and installations) with theatrical elements to present nonlinear or abstract performance works that evoke images, feelings, or references to specific moments or historical events in a manner that does not necessarily tell a cohesive story.

Choreographing Asian America is an ethnography that began in a library, rather than a studio, where in 1994 my initial catalog searches for "Asian American dance" and "Asian American choreographers" never failed to produce "zero results." "Asian American performance" did not fare any better. A search for "Asian American theater" finally yielded four publications that each offer collections of plays by Asian American writers. Three of them are anthologies: *Between Worlds: Contemporary Asian-American Plays* (1990), edited by Misha Berson; *The Politics of Life: Four Plays by Asian American Women* (1993), edited by Velina Hasu Houston; and *Unbroken Thread: An Anthology of Plays by Asian American Women* (1993), edited by Roberta Uno. In addition to these collections, James Moy's *Marginal Sights: Staging the Chinese in America* (1993) traces the historical construction of Orientalized Chineseness in the United States across a variety of representational practices, including late-nineteenth- and early-twentieth-century theater, circus acts, photography, and Hollywood film. It also includes an analysis comparing David Henry Hwang's Broadway production of *M. Butterfly* (1988) to Philip Kan Gotanda's off-Broadway production *Yankee Dawg You Die* (1988).

By the time I embarked on my fieldwork (attending rehearsals and performances with Club O' Noodles) in 1997, the first two book-length critical studies of Asian American theater had been published. Josephine Lee's *Performing Asian America: Race and Ethnicity on the Contemporary Stage* (1997) examines Asian American dramatic texts as performances of racial and ethnic identity, and finds in theatrical discourse useful metaphors for describing off-stage ethnic and racial "performances" of identity. Dorinne Kondo's ethnography *About Face: Performing Race in Fashion and Theater* (1997) deploys theatrical metaphors to discuss performances of race, ethnicity, and gender in fashion and Asian American theater. Kondo expanded the subject of Asian American theater to include the practices of watching, organizing, and writing about activities related to theatrical production.

In 1999, the publication of Yuko Kurahashi's *Asian American Culture on Stage: The History of the East West Players* provided the first historical account of Asian American theater history. Kurahashi's focus on the East West Players documents the rise of an Asian American theater movement in Los Angeles in response to the civil rights era. In this same year, Alvin Eng's *Tokens? The NYC Asian American Experience on Stage* coupled excerpts of plays and performance art pieces with interviews by new and established New York–based artists.

Adding to this growing body of scholarship is *National Abjection: The Asian American Body Onstage* (2002), Karen Shimakawa's theorization of embodiment, which positions Asian American bodies in relationship to the U.S. nation-state as abject bodies-as-subjects. Most recently, Esther Kim Lee's *A History of Asian American Theatre* (2006) accomplishes the first comprehensive introduction to the historical and theatrical contexts in which Asian American theater emerged. With the exception of *Tokens?*—which includes excerpts from multimedia dance works such as Muna Tseng's *Slut-ForArt*—the existing body of scholarship on Asian American performance focuses primarily on text-based productions.

Josephine Lee cites the problem of privileging text-based performances as an exclusionary practice that "negatively affects the publication of theater works that rely on movement, dance, or music, where the primary modes of action cannot be captured through verbal description."[2] She concentrates her study on published scripts because they are the only "fixed object[s]" that she can share with her readers, since nonliterary-based works do not lend themselves to publication.[3] A consideration of the script as a historically viable trace of live performance allows for multigenre performances that incorporate movement, dance, music, spoken text, and visual installation to be included in anthologies. For example, Muna Tseng's *SlutForArt* (1999) is described in *Tokens?* as a collaborative "visual dance-theater" and Maura Nguyen Donohue's dance *When You're Old Enough* is translated into a scripted text in *Watermark: Vietnamese American Poetry and Prose* (1998).

The inclusion of Tseng's and Donohue's dancetheater works in *Tokens?* and *Watermark,* respectively, points toward an important shift in thinking about movement-based performance in relationship to text-based plays. These initial excursions into the practice of documenting Asian American dancetheater via the written playscript raise a number of issues regarding the relationship between dancing and writing. It is not just the fact that these artists' works are translated into text that is so noteworthy—since dance historians, choreographers, and dancers have come up with multiple ways of recording dances through written descriptions and notation—but the way in which these works are translated, which does little to reveal the role of the body and of movement in the performance of the work. In other words, the physicality of the dancing body and the choreographic design of the works remain absent.

In the introduction to her script, Tseng describes *SlutForArt* as a multidisciplinary performance using prerecorded text from interviews, slide projections, and choreography, yet the textual representation of such work follows the format of a linear progression of monologues and dialogues.[4] The same is true of Donohue's *When You're Old Enough*. Absent from the scripts are a sense of Tseng's and Donohue's movement qualities and movement choices, which can provide specific, multiple, or alternate meanings, and context for spoken text. In the scripts, narration of spoken text substitutes for movement as the choreographers' primary language; whereas, any evidence of the *dancing itself* is reduced to such vague stage directions as "Dances with rosary beads"[5] and "Muna starts to dance."[6]

Dance writers have grappled with the issue of representing and/or translating bodily movement into writing in an attempt to capture, or at least reveal, dance as an ephemeral experience on the part of the spectator. As a way of resisting the reifying of dance as ephemeral, which renders it an effeminized endeavor, dance theorists such as Susan Foster (1995) have argued for the signifying capabilities of the dancing body, as well as for the necessity of attending to the material corporeality of dance—the execution of choreography. Foster also argues for consideration of the ways in which the corporeality of writers' bodies affects the translation of the dancing body into writing.[7]

To make a case for the presence of Asian American corporeality to be felt, I draw upon ethnographic research methods to understand how identity functions in both theory (disciplinary discourses) and practice (rehearsal and stage production). Borrowing from the work of Johannes Fabian (1990) and Dorinne Kondo (1997), I narrate what I call a "performative autoethnography" to think through the multiple uses of "representation" and "performance" at work in my study of Club O' Noodles. A performative autoethnography refers to the ways in which my self as a researcher, performer, and Asian American subject is created through interactions with Club O' Noodles in different contexts. My work as an active member of Club O' Noodles included both participation and observation during the rehearsal process of two major works—*Laughter from the Children of War* (1995) and *Stories from a Nail Salon* (1999).

Choreographing Asian America is a doubled ethnography, given that Club O' Noodles's performance work is itself self-reflexive about its own self-representative artistic practices. In *About Face*, Dorinne Kondo accords to performance "status as ethnographic practice, and in which ethnographies, through performance conventionally defined and through performative writing strategies, can count as theory and as political."[8] When we assign Asian American playwriting the status of ethnographic practice, we give the playwright the power to represent/re-present, rather than the traditional ethnographer. Performative ethnography locates performance itself as a form of ethnographic practice, such that the playwright/choreographer displaces the ethnographer and conducts research through art-making, even as ethnography renders the performance in question an object of study.

Kondo argues for seeing in performance the potential to challenge traditional modes of academic writing because its ephemeral nature resists textual representations. This resistance is in and of itself a form of theorization, and thus makes performance a suitable strategy for political intervention. In order to get around the problem of representing the ephemeral, Kondo locates ethnography at the site of the performance: different modes of performance become ethnographic texts that reveal information about its creators.

In doing so, she opens up the possibility of considering a variety of field sites as performance, including print advertising and her own publications, as well as her emotional responses to theatrical productions. Kondo's approach to performative ethnography provides a useful methodology for identifying and including the different stages of creating a theatrical production in a performative autoethnography.

In *Power and Performance* (1990), Johannes Fabian moves away from an *informative* ethnography—that which elicits/provides information—to that of a *performative* ethnography, which implicates the researcher in the construction of ethnographic subjects. Fabian's usage of performative ethnography investigates not only the ways in which theatrical performances provide information, but also how the information performed is created for (and by) particular situations and interactions between the ethnographer, actors, and director.[9] The social exchange between ethnographer and everyone s/he comes in contact with "gives form" to the performance of performing information. Fabian's conceptualization of performative ethnography invites the presence of the ethnographer as one who is embroiled in the process of creating meaning in relationship to the subject, and incorporates the researcher as part of the ethnographic subject.

Representation, Stereotype, Identity

Representation, stereotype, and identity are key concepts that frame my analysis of Club O' Noodles's performance work as staged self-representations of Vietnamese American identity and history. Richard Dyer (1993) defines "representation" as "[h]ow a group is represented, presented over again in cultural forms, how an image of a member of a group is taken as representative of that group, how that group is represented in the sense of spoken for and on behalf of."[10] In the 1990s, Club O' Noodles's performance work sought to confront and expose the ways in which the members viewed the necessity of the ubiquitous genre of the Hollywood Vietnam War film in order to reclaim Vietnamese American identity. The characters and themes that appear in Club O' Noodles's work speak directly to the racial stereotypes of Vietnamese and Vietnamese Americans as generated by the discourse of war. The late '70s through the early '90s saw an explosion of the Vietnam War–themed Hollywood blockbuster featuring dead or vicious Vietcong, nasty prostitutes, anonymous peasants, and oppressive jungles in such films as *The Deer Hunter* (1978), *Apocalypse Now* (1979), *Rambo* (1982), *Platoon* (1986), *Full Metal Jacket* (1987), and *Born on the Fourth of July* (1989).

The predecessors of filmic representations of Vietnamese as subhuman enemies can be found in the racist stereotypes of Asia and Asians generated by U.S. imperialism and wars fought against the Philippines (1899–1902), Japan (1941–1945), Korea (1950–1953), and Vietnam (1959–1975). Made unintelligible through foreignness, morally reprehensible through prostitution and wanton violence, and ideologically threatening through communism, after the fall of Saigon in 1975, Vietnamese subjects would remain an eternal enemy on film. As a result, the large influx of Vietnamese refugees and immigrants to U.S. shores in the late '70s and '80s was met with confusion in the American public's imagination as to who constituted an American citizen. Vietnamese refugees also presented an ideological problem for an American public already hostile to Asian immigration and, particularly, to that of an Asian population recently depicted as "the enemy." The most enduring representation of the Vietnam War is the Broadway musical *Miss Saigon* (1989), which married nineteenth-century stereotypes of Asian femininity with those of filmic discourse of the Vietnam War.

"Vietnam" signifies an era in American history that is associated with social turmoil, characterized by a failed war. The arguments about why it was a failure vary according to politico-ideological positions. Whether it failed because it was an immoral war doomed to failure or because of the American government's failure to fully support military activities in Vietnam, the experience, in the U.S. mind, remains an *American* one rather than one shared by the United States and Vietnam. Hollywood films in the 1980s depicted the Vietnam War as an event that divided American society and signaled America's loss of innocence, as if genocide of Native Americans, slavery, and legislated discrimination can be separated from the formation of the American national identity. The Vietnam War mythologized in Hollywood film focuses on that war as a series of individual injustices committed against American soldiers who are the victims of the U.S. government, war protesters, and/or the enemy Vietnamese.

Club O' Noodles's work deals specifically with mainstream representations of the Vietnam War, which are part of a repertoire of stereotypes central to American discourse about war in Asia. Renny Christopher's (1995) analysis of the Vietnam War as represented in literature draws parallels with the representation of Asia in U.S. war narratives during World War II.[11] Effeminized and infantilized, Asia is rendered childlike, immoral, and in need of guidance from a strong, sophisticated, and socially moral United States. The convoluted logic that constructs the United States as savior also posits the United States as potential victim of Asian aggression by portraying Asians as maniacal, devious, inhumane, and willing to give up their women and children to U.S. bullets in the name of an out-of-control patriotism. In claiming that Asians are always ready to sacrifice their own lives for the sake of patriotism, the U.S. military circulated an effective stereotype in order to justify the killing of Vietnamese.

Club O' Noodles is invested in dismantling this one-sided discourse of the Vietnam War by asserting that the circumstances of Vietnamese American immigration to the United States are an inextricable part of U.S. history. This is particularly relevant in a historical context: Asian immigration to the United States since the nineteenth century has generally been viewed as an invasion of opportunistic foreign aliens. Works like *Laughter from the Children of War* challenge anti-immigrant rhetoric that Vietnamese immigration, and Asian immigration in general, is an incursion against an ideal American political, economic, and cultural structure.[12] Ethnic identity is politicized in the most literal sense in order to de-aestheticize romanticized narratives of multicultural inclusionism.

Lisa Lowe's (1996) term "aestheticized multiculturalism" speaks to the practice of celebrating cultural difference within the United States, such that difference can be channeled through discourses of apoliticized authenticity. Lowe's critique of the 1990 Los Angeles Festival of the Arts identifies the way in which authentic culture and diasporic communities are collapsed in order to maintain depoliticized notions of cultural difference and authenticity. The production of a celebratory multicultural utopia situates the Asian American citizen within an awkward cultural space, where third-world artists perform "authentic" culture within a corresponding ethnic community. This type of programming suggests that both the diasporic community (the authentic participants) and the "authentic" artist must share an affinity based on an ethnic cultural heritage that is decontextualized historically and politically.[13] Club O' Noodles's performance work locates ethnicity as a politicized identity in that the work resists the formation of an ethnic-as-cultural identity in an aestheticized multicultural sense.

As a way to get into the theater, Club O' Noodles markets its performances through channels provided by aestheticized multiculturalism by identifying its own work as an expression of Vietnamese culture. Once in the theater, the label "Vietnamese American," as understood through narrow definitions of multiculturalism as "coming from somewhere else," fails to adequately describe Club O' Noodles's work. Under the rubric of multicultural rhetoric, its work has often been misinterpreted as a presentation of cultural difference rather than a critique of the conditions that create difference and otherness.

In February 1997, Club O' Noodles accepted an invitation to perform *Laughter from the Children of War* at the Bower's Museum in Santa Ana, California. The company members had agreed to perform a scaled-down, forty-five-minute version of a two-hour work, as part of a lunar New Year celebration. The organizers of the event had described the celebration to the artistic director as an open house for families and their children. Given that the museum had invited Club O' Noodles to the celebration, the company had assumed that the New Year celebration was going to be a Tet festival (Vietnamese New Year festival). Once the group arrived at the museum on the day of the performance, they discovered that they were scheduled to perform as part of a Chinese New Year celebration.

The day-long event included a program of "traditional" Chinese cultural performances—fan dances, ribbon dances, flower drum dances, Chinese orchestral arrangements, martial arts exhibits, and lion dancing—all performed by children. Each of the various youth groups, martial arts clubs, and Chinese schools represented in the program performed in rapid-fire succession. The twenty-minute version of *Laughter* was sandwiched between a fan dance and a martial arts routine.

Aside from the obvious—the fact that a Vietnamese American performance group was asked to perform during an otherwise Chinese cultural event—the event organizers failed to see the implications of their multicultural motivations. One could argue that Club O' Noodles's performance was an opportunity to critique the given situation and turn a case of mistaken identity into a political intervention. However, after the performance, the program organizer approached the artistic director about inviting the group back to the museum to present the full-length version of *Laughter*. The artistic director agreed that the group would be very interested in performing the full-length work; the museum employee responded enthusiastically with the suggestion that such a performance could be programmed in concert with an Asian food fair.

What exactly is it about a performance that explicitly addresses war, death, poverty, and racism that prompts a viewer to think about spring rolls? The museum employee's remark suggests that Club O' Noodles as a group could register as palatably multicultural (excuse the pun), while their critique remained illegible. The remark could also be read as an indication of the ways in which Club O' Noodles's critique needed to be made palatable in order to register the group's work as a multicultural event.[14]

Lisa Lowe's theory of aestheticized multiculturalism sheds light on the naturalized connection between Club O' Noodles and an Asian food fair. Without a food fair, fan dancing, and martial arts, the performing bodies in Club O' Noodles's performance work remained unreadable as properly Vietnamese. The multiculturally informed practices of programming served to contain the content of Club O' Noodles's work, thus rendering it suitable for a children's event marked as "Chinese." The New Year program included a lion dance, suggesting the presence of an "authentic-looking" and "authentic-sounding" Chinese celebration. Organizers had even invited two lion dance groups to the New Year celebration without understanding the protocol that only one should have been invited. The curators of the event viewed the lion dancers as simply "ethnic entertainers" and did not realize that both groups were highly offended upon discovering that a competing organization had been invited to perform.

The inability to recognize performers as agents of politicized aesthetics and forms demonstrates the extent to which the New Year festival and other "multicultural celebrations" are often comprised of a collection of uncontextualized, ahistoricized, and apoliticized practices. Though one of the lion dance groups left the museum in protest, event organizers did not seem concerned that a group of artists were angered enough to leave prior to a scheduled performance. The museum did not treat the transaction as a terrible loss since the remaining lion dance group would perform in two time slots instead of one. In this context, the lion dancers served as interchangeable and anonymous bodies performing a foreign and authorless dance form.

My reading of this encounter between the museum curators and Club O' Noodles attempts to expose the assumptive practice of replaceability that is common in multicultural programming. Written in the form of an ethnographic anecdote, the encounter also embodies the multifaceted ways in which representation is at work both in the encounter and in describing the encounter in writing. In returning to the concept of representation and its implications for ethnographic writing, the work of Johannes Fabian is helpful.

Fabian (1991) defines the "idea of representation" as that which requires "the prior assumption of a *difference* between reality and its 'doubles' " (emphasis in original).[15] To follow this logic is to consider representation a failing enterprise. One can then only aspire to make "better representations," or what Fabian calls "privileged representations." For Fabian, privileged representations often pass as reality. Fabian also stresses the importance of recognizing that the problem of representation does not lie in the difference between reality and its images; instead, he proposes that the problem begins with the "tension between re-presentation and *presence*." Representation is not simply a material image or object, but a process of making the "*then* into a *now*" (emphasis in original).[16] Representation is a perpetual attempt at capturing lapses in time and the act of refashioning past bodily experiences. The word "representation" encompasses the practices of creating representations, the product of representation as a praxis, and the theoretical system that allows and circulates representation as praxis and theory. Fabian calls this the practice of "representationism"—a strategy for creating and establishing ideas and systems of understanding.[17]

Fabian is likewise useful in accounting for the multiple levels of representation at work in this project. He proposes that one must think of representation as written in *response* to and not *about* the other. The other does not serve as an object of inquiry to be studied, but produces knowledge and redirects research questions. I turn to Fabian's model of performative ethnography as an impetus for finding a way to incorporate the different relationships I, as the researcher, have had in relationship to performance work, the rehearsal process, and members of Club O' Noodles, as well as to the fields of Asian American studies and dance studies at large.

At the core of this project is the relationship between Asian America and dance history. Whenever I tell people that I study Asian American dance-theater, I never fail to receive unsolicited and detailed descriptions of people's encounters with Balinese dancers, Chinese acrobats, and Japanese tea ceremonies. If the academic discipline of Asian American studies is often viewed interchangeably with Asian studies, the tendency to collapse cultures and histories is multiplied tenfold when it comes to Asian American *performance,* wherein Asian American dance is associated with something ancient, traditional, and foreign.

Edward Said (1979) characterized the practice of overculturalizing the East as in the service of empire. If, in the justification of slavery and the maintenance of colonial territories, blackness signified a visible absence of culture, the Orient symbolized culture past its prime. Scientific-sounding theories lent authority to white superiority:

> There was general agreement too that, according to a strangely transformed variety of Darwinism sanctioned by Darwin himself, the modern Orientals were degraded remnants of a former greatness; the ancient, or "classical," civilizations of the Orient were perceivable through the disorders of present decadence, but only (a) because a white specialist with highly refined scientific techniques could do the sifting and reconstructing, and (b) because a vocabulary of sweeping generalities (the Semites, the Aryans, the Orientals) referred not to a set of fictions but rather to a whole array of seemingly objective and agreed-upon distinctions.[18]

Exotic and ahistorical, the Orient served as an endless fantasy of material excess adorning an unchanging world. Aesthetic appeal provided by Orientalism was also used to justify the inassimilability of Oriental peoples. "[T]heir vices are bred in them by a civilization older than our ancient world, and there is nothing in human character on the face of this whole earth so stable, so fixed and sure and changeless, as the character of a Chinaman."[19] In the cases of the Oriental and the African, having too much or too little history is cause for moral decay.

The perception of Asians as remnants of a past civilization constructs the Asian body through the past. This is not merely a way of thinking that the body produces memory and history, but that the Asian body *is* historical rather than contemporary. The idea that the Orient is a repository of decadence underlies Orientalism, which Said deems a system of knowledge, a body of theory, and a practice that defined Europe and America through the study of difference.[20] Egypt, the Middle East, South Asia, Southeast Asia, and East Asia have all been imagined as a collapsible and consumable space called "the Orient." Not only are they interchangeable, but Orientalized cultures are consumed as highly collectible and peopleless historical objects. Since the Orient is always already "ancient," the relationship between modern-day "Orientals" and past cultures is one that is naturalized and distanced such that the "Oriental body" can be objectified and shelved. Orientalized culture can then be consumed as spiritual style.

In the United States, Asian bodily practices have been elevated to the level of superspirituality. Practices such as yoga, tai chi, and martial arts compose a middle-class alternative that allows practitioners access to spiritually or culturally "improved" lifestyles. Doing yoga suggests that one is or aspires to be enlightened, sophisticated, educated, and progressive, or demonstrates what Sarah Strauss (2005) describes as the middle-class desire to lead a better life.[21] The promise of a healthier life rooted in a non-Western practice is situated in opposition to shallow or superficial Western practices. To engage in such alternative practices allows the body to transcend the provincial and adopt a worldly and cosmopolitan knowingness outside of mainstream American culture.

Orientalism's effect on how the Asian American body is imagined in U.S. public discourse is related to that of Orientalized Asian bodily practices. In the case of Orientalized bodily practices, Asian bodies are not necessary for their continued existence. Take the cases of Ruth St. Denis, Maud Allan, and the popularity of Oriental dance at beginning of the twentieth century; white women could inhabit various "Oriental" dance forms without public acknowledgment or historical reminders of the actual Asian bodies that informed their works. St. Denis's oft-told contribution to American modern dance lay in her ability to interpret and transform Asian-ness into American-ness. In other words, Orientalism disappears Asian American bodies from the present by associating them within an imagined past that is both temporal and spatial.

The question of national belonging has been a key issue in Asian American studies in terms of the construction of Asian Americans as "perpetual foreigners" through exclusionary U.S. immigration laws. For Asian Americans, citizenship and cultural belonging in the United States has never been guaranteed, given the association of the Asian American body with an assumed past and possible foreign interests.[22] The myth of the model minority has served as the primary mode in which immigrant and native-born Asian Americans have been allowed visibility as desirable American citizens. The model-minority stereotype situates Asian Americans within the heart of U.S. democracy and capitalism by favoring highly publicized narratives of Asian immigrants who arrive in the United States with nothing and are able, within one generation, to assimilate into middle-class American lifestyles.

Such a privileging of the model-minority stereotype is grounded in Orientalist renderings of Asian subjects as a people naturally good at math and good with money.[23] The model minority disappears Asian American bodies by limiting Asian American subjectivity to narrowly defined realms of academic and economic success ascribed to Asian family structures, work ethic, and genes. The model minority serves a useful purpose, because the body of economically assimilated Asian American subjects satisfies the needs of liberal multiculturalism. The Asian American body that embodies the idea of what foreignness looks like serves up proof that the United States is a land of economic opportunity and social equality. In other words, the Asian American myth of the model minority obscures evidence of U.S. racism.

The cultural currency of the model minority as a positive stereotype, grounded in the economic terms of social assimilation through financial independence, disembodies Asian American subjects. In the introduction to his 1998 study on Asian American independent films, *Asian America Through the Lens*, Jun Xing begins by speculating on the reasons why the popularity of *Asian American* literature and *Asian* films does not translate into an equal public interest in Asian American films. He cites a friend who hypothesizes that film, unlike literature, foregrounds the visible Asian American body that the mainstream American public is unable to see. Given that representations of Asian Americans sans exotica appear mostly in the news media featuring doctors and engineers, Xing posits that mainstream film audiences are unable to imagine Asian American bodies engaged in non-Orientalized social roles.[24]

Xing's speculations about the relationship between mainstream film audiences and Asian American film offer a way to consider the relationship between the model-minority stereotype and the Asian American dancing body. The model minority as a disembodying discourse attributes Asian American success to extraordinary brainpower. Asian American critique of the myth of the model minority centers on the ways in which the myth overstates Asian American economic assimilation as evidence of a transparent ability to overcome racism aimed at racially marked bodies. To follow the logic of the model-minority myth: Asian Americans are able to "transcend" their racialized bodies by retreating to mental discipline required of academic achievement and business acumen. News reports of successful Asian American lives focus on genius or geniuslike achievements (valedictorians, child prodigies, Olympians, and rags-to-riches narratives), and not on the lives of working-class Asian Americans employed in factory work, agriculture, or menial labor—work in which the Asian American body is overly visible in racialized forms of work. This Cartesian split between the mind and the body falls along racial lines, such that Asian American bodies as the model minority are situated at one end of the spectrum of disembodiment while African Americans inhabit the other end as overly embodied subjects.

Robert Lee's *Orientals: Asian Americans in Popular Culture* (1999) historicizes the Cold War origins of the model-minority myth as a way of pathologizing the African American family in the 1960s. By decontextualizing Asian American history and emphasizing self-reliance and political silence, the myth of the model minority was used to prove that racial equality could be achieved without changing the racial hierarchy in American society.[25] The model minority is a stereotype of invisibility and draws upon Orientalist discourse without the accoutrements of the material signifiers of exotica. Asian American educational and economic successes have been attributed to traditional family structures, Confucian values, and Asian work ethics—which sounds remarkably similar to narratives of the American nuclear family, Puritanism, and the Protestant work ethic, such that the Asian American family is both socially assimilated and exoticized as foreign and atemporal.

The conflicting narratives of assimilation and exoticism within the model-minority stereotype set up an interesting set of problems for the study of Asian American performance. Through an exoticized narrative of social assimilation, the Asian American is disembodied when economic success is attributed to genetic affinity or to past tradition, rather than understanding both the socioeconomic diversity within Asian American communities and the realities of American immigration laws and patterns of immigration that create such diversity. Instead, the model minority, simultaneously, is present within the geographic borders of the United States and is ascribed to a system of ancient and foreign family dynamics. Families' culturally specific practices result in economic assimilation because they master capitalism, but this assimilation does not translate to cultural assimilation. Exoticized social assimilation removes the Asian American subject from the realm of American cultural citizenship, and thus Asian Americans remain perpetually foreign.

The model minority is not only economically assimilated, but is also a stereotype of political passivity, because it is the "properly behaved" minority. African Americans are stereotyped as complainers whose protests continually refer back to the civil rights movement, whereas model-minority success is achieved through labor in the workforce and not through political protest. In fact, Asian American political activism is generally ignored since the model-minority stereotype perpetuates the notion that Asian Americans have nothing to complain about. The internment of Japanese American citizens during World War II presents "evidence" that Asian people are not prone to political protest, even when they are mistreated. The decontextualization of this "evidence" erases Japanese American protests of the draft while they were interned, as well as the redress movement of the 1980s.

Experimental Asian American performance artists confront the stereotype of political passivity and see their work as a form of political intervention. The genesis of Asian American theater is attributed to Asian American participation in the civil rights and antiwar movements of the 1960s.[26] Yuko Kurahashi observes that the Asian American movement of the 1960s was influenced by the Black Power movement and focused on combating anti-Asian racism, on empowerment, and on finding practical solutions for ameliorating problems within the Asian American community. The emergence of Asian American protest and political action was met with the emergence of the model minority in the news media as a way to temper Asian American activism. Asian American political participation is ignored in favor of promoting the image of Asian American success based on political passivity and complacency attributed to a distinctly un-American national-as-cultural character.

As in the way that late-nineteenth-century Chinese contract labor was used as a replacement for slave labor, the model-minority stereotype positioned the laboring Asian body against black bodies. The importation of Chinese contract labor to California avoided the question of black slavery; Chinese labor represented a "lesson learned" in terms of what to do with non-white bodies once their services were no longer required. To avoid the awkward question of citizenship and birthright for descendents of enslaved Africans who remained in the United States for generations, supporters of Chinese immigrant labor created a system of legislation that prevented Chinese laborers in the United States from establishing families and producing offspring. The importation of Chinese labor in the nineteenth century proved ideal since entry into the United States was limited to able-bodied men who would later return to their families in China. Opening of U.S. doors to Asian immigrants is often construed as an act of charity on the part of the U.S. government and exists as a transitional zone between the indigenization of European immigration and slavery.

The focus on Asian American success attributed to cultural difference shifts public focus away from institutionalized racism. Robert Lee theorizes that the model-minority concept developed out of a need to restore white hegemony during economic recession, in which the financial security of the white middle-class nuclear family was undermined by the formation of a new racially gendered stereotype—the black welfare queen. In the 1980s, stories of Asian American success were used in an effort to illustrate the demise of racial inequality and thus the end of the need for the social welfare system. To avoid more blatant claims of biological difference to explain Asian American success, "Asian American" became a "culture" rather than a racial category. Pseudoscientific explanations of the Orientalized Asian body were replaced by sociological studies of Asian American "cultural difference."[27] In the 1990s, stereotypes of Asian American *culture* continued to be used as evidence to dismantle public assistance, affirmative action, and bilingual education in California.

Artists working within the genre of experimental Asian American performance attempt to disrupt the stereotype of Asian American communities as complacent entities. Club O' Noodles views its own work as an opportunity for consciousness raising and as a response to contemporary politics. Not only does it challenge the disembodiment of the model-minority stereotype by presenting Asian American bodies on stage, but they also view their productions as a form of social activism. Asian American performance challenges the supposed atemporality and ahistoricity of Asian American cultural practices in which the stereotype of the model-minority family structure stands in as an explanation of Asian American culture as a whole. Club O' Noodles borrows this domesticated narrative of the traditional-Asian-family-as-culture in their signature work, *Laughter from the Children of War* (1995), and disrupts the notion that Asian American culture (like the family) is unchanging and unresponsive to artistic and political developments.

The model minority stereotype also operates in the public imagination as a domesticating discourse that tempers Asian American masculinity. Assumed to be male, the doctor, the engineer, the accountant, and the computer nerd are figured as productive members of society who are nonthreatening. B. D. Wong plays the emotionally detached forensic psychiatrist Dr. George Huang against a cast of angry, testosterone-driven male detectives in the television drama *Law and Order: SVU*. The containment of Asian American masculinity has been used as comic relief in such films as Mickey Rooney's bucktoothed portrayal of Mr. Yuneyoshi in *Breakfast at Tiffany's* (1961), Gedde Watanabe's Long Duk Dong in *Sixteen Candles* (1984), and Mike Myer's Pitka in *The Love Guru* (2008). The gendered framing of the model minority as the sexually incompetent Asian male body stands in stark contrast to the ways in which Asian female bodies are figured in highly spectacularized sexual fantasies as prostitutes, whores, bar girls, and strippers.

Oriental Dancing Girl

One of the most recognizable Orientalist stereotypes circulating in popular culture is the Oriental dancing girl. She is appealing because of her cross-cultural sexual availability. Her profession places her outside of a protective and insular model-minority family structure. This popular representation has also been instrumental in the development of Western "high art" dance practices, and particularly in the genesis of an American high art dance tradition. The crossover appeal of the Oriental dancing girl has guided my analysis of invisible Orientalism within American dance history's narrative of artistic innovation. Invisible Orientalism is part of the larger issue in which Asian American bodies are absent from the realm of creating American national culture. The trope of the Oriental dancing girl is useful for analyzing the difficult task of seeing Asian female bodies on stage without the baggage of racially sexualized wartime prostitution.

The idea of the dancing Asian female body is doubly sexualized through Orientalist fantasies of Asian female sexual availability, as well as the suspect nature of dancing within American society in general. In addition, Asian bodily practices, aesthetics, and philosophy are simultaneously disembodied through Orientalist stereotypes of transcendence and mental discipline. Both versions of Orientalized bodily performances have informed the development of American theatrical dance since the early twentieth century. Like the model minority and narratives of exoticized assimilation, the presence of Asian aesthetics is made invisible within the history of American concert dance. This paradox of Asian aesthetics as both present and invisible in U.S. dance history is accomplished by way of Orientalist discourse, in which East and West are fundamentally different from one another.

Ruth St. Denis's early-twentieth-century Orientalist dances capitalized on American desires to see erotica—doubled via exoticism—in the form of costumes, music, stage sets, and suggestions of Oriental movement that signify the "Oriental dancing girl." St. Denis's white female body transformed the doubly exotic erotic into "art." Wrapped in the aura of Orientalism, St. Denis could dance the fantasy without being mistaken for a "real" Oriental dancing girl. Such dance scholars as Suzanne Shelton, Jane Desmond, and Sally Banes have pointed out the ways in which St. Denis did not claim authenticity in her choreography. This disclaimer would allow St. Denis to be an innovator rather than an imitator, so that her choreographic legacy can be historicized as ingenious interpretation rather than failed mimicry. These aesthetic disclaimers have created a representational bind in which "real Asian female bodies" must then function as the source from which the white women can derive sexual liberation and aesthetic inspiration.

The two most commercially successful depictions of Asian American dancing bodies employing Asian dancers, singers, and actors, *Flower Drum Song* (1961) and *Miss Saigon* (1989), deploy the three most prevalent stereotypes of Asians and Asian Americans: the model minority, war, and prostitution. Robert Lee situates the depiction of San Francisco's Chinatown and its inhabitants in *Flower Drum Song* within the Cold War origins of the model-minority stereotype.[28] Set in Vietnam, *Miss Saigon* echoes the Hollywood

Vietnam War film in its depiction of Asian women as prostitutes. These two Broadway productions form the bookends of the stereotypical ways in which the Asian American body is depicted in dance. Richard Dyer (1993) locates the power of the stereotypes in their ability to condense complex social structures and power dynamics into simple, easy-to-use formulae. However simplistic and formulaic a stereotype such as "the Oriental dancing girl" might appear, understanding the connotations of a stereotype involves an intimate knowledge of a prescribed set of social relations.

Race and Dance Studies

In challenging neoliberal paradigms of multiculturalism to account for the significance of work by Americans of Asian descent, Asian American dance history has the ability—like that of African American dance history, with its potential to bring the history of slavery into the fore of dance discourse—to bring to bear the racializing processes of invisible Orientalism into the field. The pioneering work of Brenda Dixon Gottschild, *Digging the Africanist Presence in American Performance: Dance and Other Contexts* (1996); Ann Cooper Albright, *Choreographing Difference: The Body and Identity in Contemporary Dance* (1997); Richard Green, "(Up)Staging the Primitive: Pearl Primus and 'the Negro Problem' in American Dance" (2002); Thomas De Frantz, *Dancing Revelations: Alvin Ailey's Embodiment of African American Culture* (2004); Ananya Chatterjea, *Butting Out: Reading the Resistive Choreographies through Works by Jawole Willa Jo Zollar and Chandralekha* (2004); Susan Manning, *Modern Dance/Negro Dance* (2004); and Priya Srinivasan, "The Nautch Women Dancers of the 1880s" (2009), speak to a trajectory of dance research that troubles the canon of U.S. modern dance history by questioning the racialized assumptions upon which the canon is founded.

The inclusion of colonialism and imperialism by such scholars of contemporary South Asian dance as Ananya Chatterjea, Avanthi Medhuri, and Priya Srinivasan further complicates American dance discourse on race. Priya Srinivasan's "Dancing Their Way into the Asiatic Barred Zone: Early Indian Dancers in America" (2007) elaborates on Jane Desmond's reading of Ruth St. Denis's Orientalist repertory in "Dancing out the Difference: Cultural Imperialism and Ruth St. Denis's *Radha* of 1906" (1991). By locating the effects of colonialism and racist immigration policies on early Indian dancers in the

United States between 1880 and 1907, Srinivasan is able to disrupt the ways in which Orientalism has been couched as what she calls a "benign discourse," or what I have termed as "invisible Orientalism," in dance literature.

I use the term "Asian America" to understand a process of racialization that produces the Asian American subject through immigration laws and mandatory ethnicity. Asian American subjects are never just "Asian," but are subject to mandatory ethnicity under the legal rubrics of Asian-ness as defined by the history of U.S. immigration law as applied to Asian immigrants.

Theater scholars Josephine Lee and Esther Kim Lee attend to the ways in which scholarship and programming have privileged East Asian American artists and the continued need to address the work by artists from marginalized communities within Asian America. As an initial foray into Asian American dance studies, the attempt to make Vietnamese American performance central within the literature on Asian American dance studies offers an alternative point of departure. This project adds to the existing literature on race in dance studies by further questioning the ways in which Orientalism is made invisible in U.S. dance history by focusing on Club O' Noodles, whose work makes evident the relationship between war, militarism, and the presence of Vietnamese-as-Asian-Americans in the United States.

Choreographing Asian America examines the ways in which Club O' Noodles choreographs community and identity informed by coalition politics and stereotypes circulating in high-art and middle-brow cultural productions. Given that Asian American modern and postmodern dance remains a relatively marginalized field both within cultural studies of dance and Asian American studies, research for this project took place "in the field," venturing to out-of-the-way performance venues and rehearsal spaces.

Situating this research at the intersection of Asian American cultural studies, dance history, and ethnographic writing in order to take account of the multiple ways in which Asian American bodies *choreograph* and *perform*, I investigated Asian American corporeality by attending performances, participating in rehearsals, creating performance work, and writing about past performances. A close study of performances and rehearsal processes seeks to reveal the parameters within which Asian American performance artists "choreograph" selective identities in order to align or distance themselves from each other depending on political objectives related to race, gender, sexuality, ethnicity, and/or class identifications.

This volume is organized as a performative autoethnography, each chapter providing a different entry point for understanding how the theoretical positions outlined in this introduction affect the production of contemporary Asian American performance. In tracing a body engaged in different acts of performing research, I attempt to rewrite the Asian American body back into staged and written practices of representation. A close reading of Club O' Noodles's performances and rehearsal process illuminates the creativity with which Asian American artists struggle against the conflation of race and nationality while negotiating varied degrees of personal, familial, historical, and artistic connections to Asia.

Chapter 1, "Situating Asian American Dance History," identifies the disciplinary stakes of writing an Asian American dance history within Asian American and dance studies. I use Sue Li-Jue's *Rice Women* and *The Nature of Nature* as examples of how the competing agendas of Asian American political critique and dance criticism work to narrate contradictory readings of what constitutes "successful" choreography. Li-Jue's work does not sit comfortably with Asian American (or universalized-as-white) dance critique and demonstrates the extent to which political and aesthetic expectations are shaped by disciplinary understandings of what constitutes form and content.

In defining a new area of scholarly inquiry, the question remains of how to frame Asian American dance as a practice, a cultural production, or a text. Within Asian American cultural studies, the field of literature holds such currency that literary studies and its methods for reading texts as representational practices have migrated into readings of the body. Bodies figured as texts can then be "read," so that all actions and gestures are equally deliberate and meaningful. Formulating bodies as texts can work in the case of staged performances framed as "productions"; however, there remains a blind spot in thinking through the execution and evaluation of corporeal technique. Written in two parts, chapter 1 addresses two disciplinary audiences in order to understand the radical shift of writing dance into Asian American studies and Asian America into dance studies.

Chapter 2, "Club O' Noodles's *Laughter from the Children of War,*" begins in the theater, the writing based on the conventional mode of consuming theatrical performances: sitting in a darkened theater looking out onto a proscenium stage. The spatial, temporal, and kinetic experience of watching a theatrical production translated into written text describes the performance through a close reading of both the form and the content of *Laughter.* Instead of using examples from the performance to illustrate theoretical points, chapter 2 is written from the premise that description is always already an interpretation and that performance itself provides frameworks for theorizing identity, popular culture, and representation. With an emphasis on reading choreographic forms, the analysis aims to establish the centrality of bodily movement in multidisciplinary performance that depends upon the skillfulness with which live bodies are able to manipulate and produce meaning in structured improvisations and set choreographic forms.

Moving from the theater into the rehearsal studio, chapter 3, "Rehearsing the Collective: A Performative Autoethnography," defines a methodological approach that narrates my participation in Club O' Noodles's rehearsal process. In contrast to the aesthetic and thematic content addressed in a close reading of the stage production of *Laughter*, the rehearsal process revealed a different set of concerns. Chapter 3 follows Club O' Noodles's methods for integrating new members (including myself) into the performance collective and how they train for performances. The training process destabilizes essentialized concepts of "community" as a fixed entity, since the rehearsal process is a space where the values and ideals of Club O' Noodles as a community—a refuge from racist practices of the mainstream (white) art community—are rehearsed, performed, and taught to new members.

Chapter 3 also provides context for Club O' Noodles's choice to use post-1960s' postmodern choreographic structures as aesthetic and political strategies to accommodate a transitory membership motivated by the economics of sustaining a community-based performance company. Historically, postmodern choreographic structures and movement vocabularies have been constructed as "democratic" in their radical separation of the body from social meaning. The embrace of scientific understanding of the moving body—as a collection of organs, muscles, and nerves subject to principles of weight and gravity—desexualizes the body and thus dissociates the dancing body from associations with effeminized and sexualized behavior. But when these practices are situated in a community, postmodern dance no longer functions as universal and neutral form. Club O' Noodles embodies these practices in order to call attention to the ways in which their own bodies are racialized, gendered, and sexualized.

The trajectory of this research—moving from the theater into the studio

—is interrupted by an intermission and followed by an interlude: "The Amazing Chinese American Acrobat: Choreography as Methodology." The interlude is an expanded essay based on the program notes written for a performance I created while on leave from Club O' Noodles. In 1997, Augusto Boal taught a two-week workshop at the California State University–Long Beach and Hung Nguyen was eager to have someone from Club O' Noodles attend the workshop. Since I was a full-time graduate student, I was the only person in the group who had time to attend a two-week workshop that met for four hours a day. It was during this time that I met Denise Uyehara, who had just begun teaching her Rad Asian Sisters performance and writing workshop.

Uyehara invited me to come to her workshop; my original intention was to see how Uyehara and the rest of the participants would build a grassroots Asian American feminist performance collective. The workshop was designed for participants to create and perform their own original works. Over time, I found that it became increasingly difficult to write about the Rad Asian Sisters as a group. My worry about how my own experiments would be perceived in class shifted my attention away from observing how others worked. Instead of relating to the Rad Asian Sisters as participant-observer, I took "The Amazing Chinese American Acrobat" as a hands-on opportunity to work my way through the relationship between choreography and representation. A result of a self-assigned task—make an Asian American performance—the interlude is a meditation on choreography as a research method to understand both the choreographic process of making aesthetic decisions and its attendant representational fallout.

Chapter 4, "Mapping Membership: Class, Ethnicity, and the Making of *Stories from a Nail Salon*," narrates my return to the rehearsal space with Club O' Noodles as the members prepared for a new performance project, titled *Stories from a Nail Salon*. The rehearsal process for *Stories* demonstrates the limits of Club O' Noodles's claim to represent the Vietnamese American experience, as stated in its promotional materials. Following the members of Club O' Noodles as they worked to articulate a definition of "Vietnamese American" as part of writing a mission statement for their press kit, chapter 4 demonstrates the performative nature of individual and group enunciations of Vietnamese immigrant and refugee identities.

If the analysis of *Laughter* in chapter 2 and the account of Club O'

Noodles's rehearsal process in chapter 3 impart the centrality of creating and maintaining a unified vision of Vietnamese American identity through the rhetoric of community, the question of class became a major hurdle in the making of *Stories from a Nail Salon*. The performance is based on the experiences of Vietnamese immigrants working in the nail salon industry, in which class differences among the workers themselves, and between workers and their clients, function as a source of conflict. As salon work is stigmatized as a low-class profession, Club O' Noodles took on the subject as a way to investigate the politics of exploitative working conditions and the rhetoric of the American Dream.

The premiere of *Stories from a Nail Salon* is described in chapter 5, "Writing *Nail Salon*." My participation in the rehearsal process involved assisting as rehearsal director, as well as choreographing and performing sections of the piece. The result is a fragmented description, because I was unable to see the performance in its entirety. In addition, I saw much of the performance from backstage, and the final videotaped recording of the work is composed of footage from multiple performances, resulting in a piece in which different performers appear in the same role from scene to scene. My corporeality "gets in the way" of representing *Nail Salon* in its totality, and reveals the limits of privileging corporeal knowledge. The chaos of last-minute substitutions and the resulting performances demystify the glamour of improvisation and the adaptability of the performing body.

Chapter 6, "Pedagogy of the Scantily Clad: Studying *Miss Saigon* in the Twenty-first Century," launches the reader back into the mainstream theater to revisit *Miss Saigon* nearly a decade after the megamusical closed on Broadway. Six years after *Miss Saigon* premiered in London, it opened in Los Angeles at the Ahmanson in 1995. Angered and dismayed by the musical's reduction of the Vietnam War to a series of recycled clichés, Hung Nguyen began work on *Laughter* in response to the critical acclaim and sold-out audiences for *Miss Saigon*. The musical closed on Broadway in 2001, around the same time that Hung Nguyen stepped down from his directorship of Club O' Noodles.

Chapter 6 examines how Club O' Noodles's critique of *Miss Saigon* (as described in chapter 2) continues to resonate, and considers the touring version that has reached major and regional theaters throughout the United States, Europe, and Asia. The impact of the resurrected musical has surpassed that of the original. In the 1990s, *Miss Saigon* existed under a cloud of controversy over the casting of white actor Jonathan Pryce in a role written for a Eurasian character, and the musical's racist retelling of the Madame Butterfly narrative set during the Vietnam War. The twenty-first-century version exists outside of the musical's controversial past and has managed to escape readings of its racist, sexist, and imperialist content. Instead, the musical is now marketed as an example of artistic survival and political acumen, with the added bonus of claiming educational value as an accurate, albeit theatricalized, history of the Vietnam War. Chapter 6 compares the stage version of *Miss Saigon* with its accompanying educational curriculum to understand how the production manages to appropriate the very kinds of Asian American critique proposed in the performance work of Club O' Noodles.

To disallow *Miss Saigon* from having the last word (as it seems unlikely that the musical will ever go away), the epilogue ends with a reading of Maura Nguyen Donohue's *Lotus Blossom Itch* as an example of choreography that parodies the history of Orientalism in U.S. modern dance history and points toward new possibilities for what the Asian American body can articulate through dance.

1

SITUATING ASIAN AMERICAN DANCE STUDIES

To understand the disciplinary stakes in terms of what it means to write about dance in the context of Asian American studies and Asian America in dance, this chapter begins with an analysis of Sue Li-Jue's *Rice Women* (2000) and *The Nature of Nature* (2001). Questions of aesthetics, questions of politics, and questions of the pleasures of watching dancing bodies all come together in Sue Li-Jue's self-described "Asian American dance company"; her work offers an opportunity to reflect upon conflicting definitions of what constitutes "good art" and "good politics" within dance and Asian American studies. To propose a model for theorizing Asian American dance, the rest of the chapter investigates the relationship between art and politics in a two-part narrative—(1) Locating Dance in Asian American Studies and (2) Locating Asian America in Dance—to situate the particular ways in which both dance and Asian America are marginalized sites of inquiry in relationship to each other.

The program notes for the September 29, 2000, performance of Facing East Dance and Music's production of *Rice Women* (2000) describe the company's work as "expressed through modern dance with an Asian aesthetic." The premiere of Sue Li-Jue's evening-length work featured an ensemble of Asian American women working in a Limon-Humphrey modern dance vocabulary punctuated by Li-Jue's signature barrel turns. The dancers' bodaies were athletic, fluid, precise, and articulate as they executed the different sections of Li-Jue's choreography that depicted, reflected upon, or embodied the experiences of Asian American women past and present—a present including that very moment of dancing itself.

In an interview, Li-Jue, the artistic director of the company, pointed out that reviews of *Rice Women* focused the majority of their comments on a two-minute section of her choreography that offered what she thought was an easy-to-read critique of stereotypical representations of Asian female sexuality.[1] This section of an evening-length work featured Li-Jue's all—Asian American female dance company performing as a group of stiff-jointed dancing dolls dressed identically in glittery magenta wigs, short shorts, and tank tops. The dancing doll as a symbol of female subjugation has been a recurring role in Western concert dance since the late nineteenth century. In Arthur Saint-Léon's *Coppélia* (1870) and Michel Fokine's *Petrouchka* (1911), the role of the dancing doll as a nonsentient object makes visible the interchangeability of desire for live female bodies with that of mechanical bodies that magically come to life. The dolls are novel in that they can be "turned on" to move in public, but their real worth is their ability to come to life in the privacy of libidinal dreams. Dr. Coppelius believes his doll has come to life in what he thinks is the privacy of his workshop; and Petrouchka, alone in his room, away from the crowd at the fair, anguishes over the dancing ballerina doll. In Marius Petipa and Lev Ivanov's *The Nutcracker* (1891), Clara's nutcracker, a gift from the mysterious uncle/family friend/party guest, turns into a prince who escorts her into a romantic, preadolescent dreamworld.

Accompanied by a poem about China dolls and other infantilizing terms, Li-Jue's dancing dolls do the additional work of confronting racialized mechanisms of control over and desire for Asian women and girls. Li-Jue herself appeared on stage in the persona of a young girl playing with a stack of identical blond Barbie dolls while the chorus of "live dolls" returned to dance behind her. This was a humorous and witty critique of the ways in which Asian American girls and women are gendered and sexualized through mass media and consumerism—and, as Li-Jue pointed out, the reviewers "got it."

"Getting it" has long been the bane of modern dance and its audiences. It is at the historical root of the antagonistic relationship between the belief that dance is supposed to act as a universal language and the not-uncommon perception of modern dance as inaccessible. Which is why I was so surprised when Li-Jue complained that the reviewers got it. Li-Jue's point of contention was that reviewers focused their attention on the short but funny Barbie doll section of the dance and failed to write anything substantial about longer sections of what she considered complex choreography. According to Li-Jue, with the exception of the Barbie doll dance, she and her company spent months working on the choreography that comprised most of the evening-length performance. Li-Jue claimed that she and her dancers threw the two-minute Barbie doll dance together in fifteen minutes and, even though reviewers and audience members alike found it highly entertaining and politically successful, she would not do it again.

True to her words, Li-Jue's next work, *The Nature of Nature,* premiered in March 2001 at the Asian Pacific Cultural Center in Oakland, California, and offered something entirely different. Based on the Chinese theory of the five elements—earth, metal, wood, water, and fire—Li Jue cast five Asian American women, each dancing the role of one element. She choreographed a solo for each element that drew inspiration from the colors, emotions, actions, ideas, and places associated with it. Unlike in *Rice Women,* there were no Barbie dolls, no depictions of grandmothers playing mahjong, and no references to immigration, alienation, or oppression.

In her review of *The Nature of Nature* that appeared in the *San Francisco Bay Guardian*, Sima Belmar accused Li-Jue of perpetuating stereotypes. Belmar described the costumes, visual installations, and set design in great detail and even quoted directly from the text that accompanied the dancing. In fact, she had something to say about the entire performance except for the dancing itself. She wrote:

> The dancers of Facing East are all beautiful movers. But the piece relied so heavily on the costumes, set, sound, and unexamined text, that the choreography looked like a lazy afterthought, one that might stir you from sleep, but not enough to get you out of bed. Stripped of its accoutrements, would there have been a dance at all? . . . Facing East cites as its mission to present work that explores being Asian American and female. Thus far Li-Jue has done little more than serve up weakly ironic takes on stereotypes and slurs for our collective.[2]

Belmar laments the absence of an identifiable critical edge in Li-Jue's choreographic vision of what it means to be Asian American and female. If this is the case and Li-Jue's danced answer is insufficient, then what is such an exploration of Asian American women supposed to look like? What does a critic like Belmar see as lacking in Li-Jue's choreographic answer? What does the work not do, when the audience is so close to the five Asian American women on stage that one can see and hear the breath pattern needed to barrel through space?

Working primarily in a Humphrey-Limon movement vocabulary, Li-Jue's choreography is situated clearly within a modern dance aesthetic that might be described as luscious and leggy modern dance. It is an aesthetic that requires a body versed in the logic of classical ballet lines, coupled with a flexible torso and a willingness to shift one's center line. Her conscious incorporation of an "Asian" aesthetic does not lie in the movement vocabulary but in her collaboration with an experimental taiko ensemble, set designers, costumers, and dancers. In *The Nature of Nature*, Asian and Asian American—ness appear as both form and authorship. She is Asian American, her dancers are Asian American, the musicians are Asian American, the set designer is Asian American, and the costume designer is Asian American. Her collaborators incorporate "Asian forms" into their compositions and set designs; however, Li-Jue herself does not.

If in *Rice Women* the inclusion of an Asian Americanist critique makes an exploration of Asian American—ness visible, does the lack of such an inclusion in *The Nature of Nature* render the exploration invisible? Li-Jue's collaboration goes unrecognized as an Asian Americanist move as *The Nature of Nature* fails to illuminate Asian American experiences when examined under a sociological lens. In other words, the way in which Li-Jue uses "Asian aesthetics" through her collaborative efforts in the absence of irony proves uncomfortable to watch since it teeters on the edge of autoexoticism.[3] The Asian American cultural critic wants such autoexoticism to be sarcastic, campy, ironic, parodic, or at least to be performed by children or "regular" community people as part of a "multicultural cultural experience." As it stands, aesthetics and abstraction remain elusive topics for Asian American artists when their work is expected to offer some sort of overt sociological analysis or function as evidence of a socially conscious form of roots-type Asian-ness.

Let us look again at Li-Jue's choreography. The dancers are stunning in their athleticism. The woman dancing the role of Fire in *The Nature of Nature* is wearing a miniature red outfit with pompoms on her head. She darts mischievously through the taiko drums, steals a pair of drumsticks for herself, and plays with the band. Definitely modern dance with an Asian twist, but is it *just* modern dance with an Asian twist? It has been a long-held practice to allow Asian American artists the ability to merge Eastern forms and themes into the modern dance idiom, as long as these experiments do not appear to be the universally applicable movement vocabularies of modern dance training. Within the logic of modernist understandings, Li-Jue's modern dance experiments can only be innovative on the level of theme, whereas the choreography goes unnoticed even as the dancing itself is made visible by visibly Asian American bodies.

The reactions to Li-Jue's work and Li-Jue's subsequent response illustrate the multiple registers that articulating an "Asian American dance history" must attend to. From an Asian Americanist point of view, Li-Jue fails or refuses to articulate an overtly critical politics, while the aesthetics of her choreographic practice go unseen. From a dance point of view, Li-Jue can never occupy a central position within modern dance if modernist investments in aesthetics refuse to see the politics of how racialized bodies are cast within discourses of universality.

Locating Dance in Asian American Studies

The study of Asian American cultural practices has largely been concerned with the representation of Asian Americans in mainstream U.S. culture and the recognition of Asian American self-representational practices. In Asian American theater studies, Josephine Lee, Dorinne Kondo, and Karen Shimakawa look to theater as a cultural site, like that of film or literature, where Asian American playwrights negotiate their relationship to citizenship, personal and social history, and agency. As Esther Kim Lee observes, the majority of Asian American theatrical works that have been studied are text-based plays performed in a naturalistic style. She attributes this to a history in which many of the Asian American theater artists who began working in the 1960s modeled their theater companies on U.S. regional theater in terms of repertory.[4]

To create acting opportunities, companies like East West Players in Los Angeles, California, produced mainstream musicals that featured all–Asian American casts in non–Asian American roles. These companies also provided an important venue for nurturing the creation of new works that featured Asian American stories and characters.[5] To combat the over-the-top stereotypes of Asians and Asian Americans on stage and screen, the theatrical convention of telling stories in a naturalistic mode would make for a powerful tool in the retelling of Asian American history and subjectivity. J. Lee refers to these plays as "family stories," in which the lives of Asian Americans are portrayed in mundane terms of everyday life. Plays written and performed in English allow Asian American characters to tell a legible story and demystify foreignness.

The vocabulary of abstract movement poses a difficult challenge in the retelling of Asian American stories. Unlike the ways in which dance has been written into diasporic African cultural history—as a mode of resistance to slavery, Jim Crow laws, the civil rights movement, and institutional racism—there is no pan–Asian American discourse about the role of dance in Asian America. There are specific instances in practices, like hula, Pilipino Cultural Night productions, and the revival of Khmer dance in western Massachusetts, in which discourses of survival and resistance toward cultural imperialism exist; however, the conditions of resistance are unique to each form's history. As a whole in the United States, Asian dance evokes something more pleasant than political resistance. It speaks to aestheticized notions of heritage in the form of either folk dance, as in the case of the ubiquitous fan dance featured at Chinese New Year's celebrations, or classical tradition, as in the case of Bharata Natyam performed for second-generation Indian girls' *arangetrams* (the classical Indian dancer's first solo performance). Although the forms might be products of political resistance, they are not perceived as such by the general public.[6]

The absence of dance from Asian American studies speaks to larger issues about dance in relationship to the structure of the academy at large. In her history of theater studies, Shannon Jackson attempts to understand the historical forces that both include and marginalize theater and performance studies in the U.S. academy. At the core of her argument, Jackson identifies the ways in which "theory" comes to power as a defensive response to the unstable role of the humanities in increasingly corporatized universities.

Jackson locates much of this anxiety within the humanities, in English and literature departments under pressure to justify and identify objects of study. As a result,

> the profession of literature has served as the primary vehicle for establishing the cultural capital of modern English-speaking universities and, hence, has also served as the barometer for gauging the legitimacy of other humanistic fields. . . . Literature and English depart-

ments have produced some of the most significant and widely circulated critical paradigms in the humanities, models and frameworks
that many drama, theatre, and performance studies have adopted
despite their own anti-literary rhetoric and institutional location.[7]

Theater studies, with its proximity to *theater* as a bodily practice, functions in
a gendered relationship to literature such that the disavowal of practice and
the adoption of literary methods of analysis masculinizes theater studies.

For this reason, the stakes for claiming dance within Asian American
studies are high. Since Noverre's attempts to recuperate dance from the
bottom of the professional hierarchy at the Academy Royale de la Musique
and Danse in the eighteenth century, dance continues to sit at the bottom of
the academic hierarchy. Aware that dance studies have been feminized in
relationship to music and theater, dance scholars such as Susan Foster attempted to bring the subject of dance into academic discourse in the 1990s by
speaking in the language of literary scholarship.[8]

Even though Asian American studies takes up an oppositional space
within the U.S. academy, the field replicates disciplinary hierarchies. Within
Asian American studies, literature, history, sociology, and anthropology constitute core disciplines of study. Because of Asian American cultural studies'
emphasis on literary analysis, it has become the primary mode of analyzing
Asian American artistic practices. In other words, performance is made
visible through the proliferation of scholarly studies, regardless of how marginalized the actual practice of performance remains within the physical
spaces of the discipline.

It is no secret in the Asian American performance art community that
ethnic studies programs, Asian American studies programs, and Asian Pacific Islander student organizations in U.S. colleges and universities operate
as a touring circuit for Asian American performers looking for venues to
present their work. This realm of presenting opportunities is often referred
to informally, and in some cases disparagingly, as "the college circuit." On
college campuses, established artists like Denise Uyehara, Jude Narita, Dan
Kwong, 18 Mighty Mountain Warriors, Here and Now, and TeAda Productions have found a receptive audience for artistic works that embody
the ideas espoused by contemporary Asian American and ethnic studies
scholarship.

Since the publication of Dorinne Kondo's *About Face,* Josephine Lee's *Performing Asian America,* Karen Shimakawa's *National Abjection,* Yuko Kurahashi's *Asian American Culture on Stage*, and Esther Kim Lee's *A History of Asian American Theater*, live theatrical production has entered into the discourse of Asian American studies as a relevant field of study alongside literature, history, and sociology. What differentiates live performance from these other fields in terms of its relationship to Asian American studies is the physical proximity between practitioners (the performers) and their audiences (scholars/students/the academy). Asian American dance and performance art require the physical space provided by the academy to be seen; and the concepts and analytical frameworks generated by Asian Americanists in the academy make the work by Asian American artists legible in history. At the same time, scholars depend on artists to create the subjects of study as well as examples to back up their theoretical assertions.

The political orientation of work such as Club O' Noodles's *Laughter from the Children of War* and *Stories from a Nail Salon* is typical of artists who can tour the university circuit successfully. Shared political agendas with Asian American studies, such as consciousness raising in matters of oppression and discrimination, allow live performances on college campuses to function as another mode—like literature, history, and sociology—of dispelling stereotypes, promoting visibility, articulating political concerns, and educating the public on Asian American issues.

In this context, the politically attuned performance operates as the last bastion for overturning the "model minority" that so often haunts the subject of Asian Americans and education. Incursions into performance art represent a rebellion against stories of Asian Americans who raise grading curves, become class valedictorians, and win Olympic medals, as depicted in Hollywood film and television. If the myth of the model minority disembodies the Asian American subject as a politically passive cultural outsider, then the myth, and thus desire, for the performing body holds the promise of enacting visible resistance to dominant paradigms of Asian racialization in the United States.

Dancing—that activity associated with tight clothes, too much skin, too much makeup, and recreation—is an embarrassing activity that is also a site of desire. As in the film *Shall We Dance?* (2004), the desire for consuming dance is a guilty pleasure to be hidden away as if it is something too embar-

rassing to admit to. This tension between desire for dance and embarrassment for that desire is driven by the mystique of dance in contemporary U.S.
culture. Dance holds a seductive sway over the imagination as visually embodied practice shrouded in the possibilities of high art, cultural avant-
gardism, beauty, radical politics, voyeurism, and ultimately—stardom.

The idea of dancing and the image of "the dancer" are in themselves
fantasies upon which additional fantasies of alternative identities and the
promise of bodily transformations are superimposed. Live performance as an
idea stirs up desires of wanting *to see,* which is then sublimated into wanting
to be, the body on stage.[9] This love of dance is often used to explain the
expectation and willingness of unemployed dancers to rehearse and perform
for free, well beyond the definition of internship or volunteer work, as a way
to "get in the door."

Dance as the object of both desire and denigration effeminizes dance
within the academy and U.S. culture at large. The effeminization of dance is
replicated within Asian American disciplinary discourse. As in the case of
Sue Li-Jue's work, for dancing to be legible, it must entertain and be in the
service of politically expedient ideas; otherwise, it is a frivolous or lazy after-
thought. Feared, worshipped, and dismissed, live performance as a practice is
not necessarily viewed as a specialized activity in itself.

I must bring up these problematic responses to Asian American performance in the context of Asian American studies. Although there is no doubt
that the programming of performance by the academy provides some artists
needed visibility, this trend is problematic when performance is viewed as a
cure-all for the doldrums of academic conferences. In other cases, the field
looks to the arts to expand its visibility—and performance becomes the "cool-
est" way to do this.

This visibility offered to performance within Asian America is mislead-
ing. Universities like to publish photographs of dance class in order to project
cultural sophistication and breadth; however, it is not uncommon for dance
to be marginalized on university campuses in terms of resources. Performance is often used as the celebration tacked on at the end of conferences and
heritage weeks. Too many times, conference organizers invite artists to perform as part of conference panels, without the recognition of art-making as
full-time work, and give no thought to paying an artist. Or performance
serves as a relaxing epilogue to shore up the day's "real" presentations (read,

"papers") and keynote speeches. I often find it amazing how the most serious Asian American cultural critique becomes starry-eyed when faced with performance, and how even scholars are unable to see past theatrical clichés, viewing performance as a more entertaining way to receive the same message delivered by the "real" scholars and activists.

Live performance takes up a conflicted space within Asian American studies. Scholars herald it as either the absolute act of political and social rebellion or the purest form of reclaiming cultural heritage, at the same time as they easily dismiss it as lightweight activism. Alternatively, performance might stand in as the public face of activist work. Performance is evidence that Asian American talent has arrived on the cultural scene, but it is seldom taken seriously as a discipline. While literature and social protest represent the constant voice of Asian America, performance exists as celebration—living proof of Asian American activism, but quickly set aside as a diversion to the real tasks of studying literature, economics, and social activism.

What kind of audience do these conditions generate? I ask because Asian American critique of Asian American performance is often a championing of radical political ideals without regard to artistic innovation; the same type of critique occurs in mainstream art communities that view Asian American contemporary dance solely through a sociological lens. It is true that many Asian American performance artists do address issues of racism, sexism, and other forms of social oppression, but it is still a disservice to evaluate such work purely on content without consideration of form.

In a conversation with performance artist Denise Uyehara, she identified the problem of "reinventing the wheel" within Asian American performance —in which artists of color are always "emerging" and "the first," even if they have been touring the same work for years. I think it is important to link this to the marginalization of Asian American performance within the mainstream art world, in which academia provides a platform as a fallback touring opportunity. I do not mean to disparage the college touring circuit, but to emphasize the particulars of this audience. Accompanying the increasing interest in Asian American studies on college campuses in the United States is a ready-made audience. Comprised primarily of eighteen- to twenty-two-year-olds, campus audiences are renewable every four years. The majority of these students who develop an interest in Asian American studies have come to define themselves as Asian American. Highly educated and working in an academic social milieu, this audience is invested in seeing public performances or enunciations of Asian American identity.

It is also important to take note of the fact that it is an audience that on the whole does not regularly attend live theatrical productions. The average Asian American college student attending an Asian American performance may realize several new experiences simultaneously. It might be the first time s/he has ever attended a live theatrical performance, the first time s/he has ever seen an Asian American person on stage, and/or the first time s/he has ever seen a performance that deals specifically with the experience of being an Asian American person. As a result, Asian American performance art is often compared to and contextualized as an alternative to Hollywood film and television representations, rather than performance techniques or traditions that an artist is trained in or is drawing from.

Performance work that deals with themes of oppression, the public portrayal of the specificity of Asian American experiences, and the insistence on Asian American hipness validates a project of continuous consciousness-raising that occurs within an undergraduate academic setting. Oftentimes artists feel trapped by needing to perform identity through explicit performances of oppositional representations that spell out their politics to Asian American audiences invested in defining an Asian American consciousness. Denise Uyehara considers her signature work, *Hello (Sex) Kitty* (1994), an easy sell on college campuses since it clearly defines her as a queer Asian American woman who is reclaiming her sexuality. References to herself as the first and only Asian American lesbian stand-up comedian, and to Hello Kitty, Kabuki, and the *Joy Luck Club*, draw on recognizable images found in Hollywood film and mall culture. Because this piece directly confronts specific Orientalist stereotypes as its thematic focus, audiences can identify the work as critique of racism, sexism, and homophobia.

Uyehara's *Maps of City and Body* (1999) also deals with issues of gender, sexuality, and bodily identity. On the surface, "Denise Uyehara" as a name holds marketing power as it symbolizes the promise of a queer, feminist, and Asian American performance. Unlike *Hello (Sex) Kitty*, presentations of *Maps of City and Body* have been met with the confused reply, "Which part of the show was Asian American?" Without the obvious critiques of racial stereotypes and archetypal Asian American childhood memories, her work becomes unidentifiable in terms of inhabiting a thematic Asian American niche. The confused reaction to the work signals the powerful expectation that thematic content alone satisfies political expectation. An artistic experiment that does not have an explicitly identifiable theme is under suspicion. It can be considered less "political" by Asian Americanists, and therefore not politically progressive enough to be characterized as an example of Asian American self-representation.

How then does one talk about aesthetics, or, more importantly, find a language to discuss Asian American cultural production without committing the same crime as mainstream (white) criticism by reducing it to a matter of political progressiveness and historical catch-up? There is a gap between Asian-America-as-political and modernist understandings of artistic consumption. To be considered an enlightened dance spectator unencumbered by the weight of racialized, gendered, or classed bodies requires one to attend Merce Cunningham's performances of abstract chance procedure and computer-generated choreography year after year at Berkeley's Zellerbach Hall. Of course, having seen a recent exhumation of *Summerspace* (1958) is a matter of possessing a particular brand of cultural capital—one that supercedes cultural specificity predicated on national borders. In this case "cultural" signifies culture with a capital *C,* and the consumption of Culture is the knowing of how to consume pure aesthetics, no matter how dated the Robert Rauschenberg screen-printed unitards look or John Cage's music sounds. Participating in Culture is to be a cosmopolitan and cultureless (deracinated, nonethnic, and ungendered) subject. With such opposing and understood conditions of culture/Culture, how is it possible to discuss the Asian American body and Asian American choreography outside the parameters of sociological evidence or reverting to nostalgic references to a "natural/essential" Asian body?

For this reason I believe that it is important to look at Asian American performance not as the bounded entity presented some evening at a particular time, but as a social space in which Asian American artists are grappling with questions of form, content, and process as markers of identity. This approach may serve to tackle some of the issues that Josephine Lee points to as problematic in her own study of Asian American drama.[10] Lee posits that the limitations of her own study are symptomatic of a systematic exclusion of what is considered Asian American performance. One such exclusion is what she identifies as a lack of access to or unavailability of dramatic works in the form of published texts. The focus on lack of accessibility to Asian American performance via dramatic texts in a published form creates an automatic crisis in terms of defining what constitutes Asian American theater or performance.

There are a significant number of Asian American performance artists whose work does not fall into a narrow category of "published play texts." In an attempt to define a not-yet-defined field of work, Josephine Lee's focus on published play texts inadvertently relegates the body that is central to live performance to a secondary role. Performing on stage as a bodily activity is oftentimes overlooked by textual analyses of scripted dialogue. Lee's study of Asian American dramatic texts interrogates the ways in which playwrights tackle issues of identity and representation. She identifies the significance of Asian American theater as a body of work that is a conscious attempt to re-present the Asian American body in a public space. The idea of the visible and public body is an important point to focus on since Asian American performers work in a cultural environment that still finds it difficult to "see" Asian bodies outside narrow stereotypes—one of which is absence.

In order to examine the significance of seeing Asian bodies in America, one must look at Asian American performance as something that does not exist solely within the confines of the written text. It is important to examine the "unpublished" and "inaccessible" work to find the bodies that challenge homogenizing scholarly practices. This is a way not only to solve Josephine Lee's problem of what she calls "unavailability," but also to call attention to the larger question of genre. The fact that many contemporary artists of color use postmodern techniques of combining text, bodily movement, and visual imagery to create work can provide a different perspective for understanding the difficulty of finding published texts. These choreographic techniques do not translate easily into a publishable play text, and this genre precludes the possibility of separating a discussion of the body of the performer, the performance, and recorded traces of the performance from any text that may be included in the work.

Because of the great disparities in funding practices, programming, and accessibility to resources—and in order to compensate for the lack of published play texts and to broaden scholarly sources—it is important to consider searching out obscure theaters to watch one-night productions. Venue affects the way in which Asian American performance is seen and defined. Access to particular types of performance space contributes to the aesthetic development of Asian American performance. There is a close connection between the development of Asian American studies and student activist groups and the circulation of performance. While academic departments and student groups can be effective at and enthusiastic about drawing an audience for performance events, there tends to be a shortfall when it comes to technical support for artists. Because of a lack of communication between ethnic studies and performing arts departments, performances are scheduled by students who do not necessarily have access to adequate or appropriate performance space, lighting, and other technical needs.

Asian American performance generates interest within academia through department- or student-sponsored performance events. Since students may be seeing live theater and Asian American performers for the first time, the circumstances in which a performance piece is presented affect the way in which aesthetics develop. While touring with Club O' Noodles, I witnessed the group adapt their work for spaces that ranged from proscenium stages of varying sizes to multipurpose rooms with no designated stage areas. The absence of lighting and other theatrical infrastructure, as well as carpeted floor surfaces, required performers to edit their performances for each space. The infrastructure of performance spaces affects more than just the timing and spacing of bodies on stage. Having to make drastic decisions to leave out sections or stage sets dramatically affects the aesthetic impact of a performance piece both figuratively and literally.

If the appeal of seeing Asian American performance lies in the promise of seeing a live Asian body on stage, it is imperative to rewrite the body back into Asian American performance studies. Josephine Lee argues that the significance of the Asian body on stage lies in its capacity as a potentially threatening signifier of power. But what exactly does the body *do* on stage in order to accomplish this? I assert that the political potential of Asian American performance depends upon a refiguring of the ideology under which Asian bodies are visually perceived. In order to identify performance as a tactical move, one must avoid draining the body of its agency, otherwise the "body" becomes a collection of physical markers defined as "Asian American" rather than a thinking agent in the process of creating history in the moment for the future. It is important to pay attention to bodily actions because the physicality of the performer reveals complex relationships between the body and its environment. To consider the body also reveals the ways in which the category of "artist" is romanticized as the rebellious individual who becomes an appropriate symbol for collective interests.

Audiences (both theoretical and physical) are a significant factor for an artistic community built around the idea that there is an "Asian American community" and dependent upon the notion that there is an audience that identifies itself as such. One must also consider the relationship between performance and an audience invested in "seeing itself" within Asian American performance, and viewing performance as an extension of political agendas developing in Asian American studies as an academic discipline. As Sue Li-Jue herself demonstrates, the issue of "getting it" is in reality a backstage obsession that should not be dismissed.

Locating Asian America in Dance Studies

If dance holds such a conflicted space between desire and denigration within Asian American studies, what are the stakes for claiming Asian America within modern dance? If Asian American theatrical performance is an alternative site for self-representation, what does it mean to write about Asian American performance within a history of a genre (modern dance) that also sees itself as a self-reflexive and alternative cultural practice? If ballet in the United States in its most codified and institutionalized form can be culturally marginalized, modern dance is even more so as it attempts to work out multifaceted relationships between the body that dances with agency and the body seen dancing.[11] Locating Asian America within modern dance requires not only the undoing of canonical dance history, but also the recognition that dance already holds a fragile place within U.S. cultural history at large. In practice, the claim for dance as a meaningful endeavor is never a given and is one that dance scholars must continually insist upon, in much the same way that Asian American studies is situated against mainstream disciplines like literature, history, and sociology.

It is no wonder that I had almost given up writing about dance in the weeks following the terrorist attacks in New York City and Washington, D.C., as growing numbers of casualties were reported in the news. I found myself succumbing to the feeling that the state of the world had little to do with dance, when I came across a full-page newspaper advertisement for the

Pennsylvania Ballet's annual production of *The Nutcracker*.[12] The photographer captured a male dancer performing the role of Tea, suspended in midair with his legs hyperextended at the apex of a perfect 180-degree, second-position *grand jeté*. Tea is dressed in a green and yellow, pajamalike satin costume; his eyes are drawn into exaggerated slants. Glued to his chin and upper lip is the iconic, long and stringy Fu Manchu–style facial hair. This photograph captured the depth to which Orientalism is ingrained in U.S. culture, such that the offensiveness of a yellow-face caricature could go unnoticed by the company, and serve as an advertisement for its biggest money-making production of the year.

This *Nutcracker*'s Tea character, and so many others like it, serves as a glaring reminder of how U.S. culture is unable to recognize how twenty-first-century Orientalism is a form of racism identical to its nineteenth-century predecessor. U.S. racial discourse evaluates race relations in terms of economic equality, legislated civil rights, and the presence of visually different people within its national boundaries, and to a certain extent representation within mass media and popular culture. But, for some reason, images such as Tea's are excused as inconsequential entertainment because they circulate within the realm of feminized and, in the case of ballet, infantilized high art dance practices. Associated with women, female children, sexually suspect men, and the rhythmic propensities of dark-enough-skinned people, dance—like the Orientalized Asian body—is marginalized in U.S. culture as an apolitical and culturally dispensable entity. If dancers, choreographers, critics, and scholars seek to make a case for the importance of dance in a continuously hostile artistic and economic environment, we must insist on examining our inherited practices. As dance scholars, it is not enough to promote and celebrate. If we want dance to be taken seriously, and in order to understand its full power, impact, and relevance to society, we must face the full extent to which dance participates in creating the conditions of the cultures we live in.[13]

Repeatedly, Asian American activists and scholars have argued for the inclusion of Orientalism as part of the U.S. discourse on race relations. Critiques of U.S. race relations have focused primarily on black/white racial conflicts. The enslavement of African peoples, Jim Crow laws, and the lynching of African American men have been domesticated as defining contradictions between U.S. democratic ideals and discriminatory legislation. The racial agenda set forth by Orientalism is harder to identify since the United States maintains and regulates non-white and non-black racial discrimination through immigration laws and foreign wars. While racism is viewed as a domestic social problem between people who should be equal based on the legislated guarantees of citizenship, Orientalism is not viewed as a racist project. Under the general rubric of "cultural differences," Orientalism is viewed as an unavoidable and expected problem between nations. Orientalism is further deterritorialized from the United States through the simultaneous process of patrolling national borders for foreign bodies while celebrating faraway cultures. Depoliticized by "sincere" research, dance historians fail to recognize the clout of Orientalism. Instead, historians of U.S. modern dance mistake Orientalism as simply a matter of artistic sensibility, in much the same way that Negrophilia and Primitivism have been understood in European art. In 1979, Edward Said wrote:

> Thus a very large mass of writers, among whom are poets, novelists, philosophers, political theorists, economists, and imperial administrators, have accepted the basic distinction between East and West as the starting point for elaborate theories, epics, novels, social descriptions and political accounts concerning the Oriental, its peoples, customs, "mind," destiny and so on.[14]

If we add "dance" to this list, we as dance scholars can no longer hide behind the academic stigma as purveyors of frivolous endeavors. The example of Tea demonstrates that even to begin locating Asian America within dance, one must start by unearthing the depth of U.S. modern dance history's entanglements with Orientalism. In doing so, one can start to see how Asian and Asian American bodies both past and present are hidden and obscured behind the white, female, middle-class, dancing bodies that take up center stage in the formation of canonical histories.

We need to look at how our failure to engage in the reexamination of Orientalism is a failure to account fully for the impact that dance has on society. Jane Desmond's 1991 analysis of Ruth St. Denis's 1906 *Radha* and Amy Koritz's 1997 analysis of Maud Allan's 1908 *Vision of Salome* begin critical discussions that call attention to white European and U.S. women's identification with Orientalist imagery in an effort to articulate new models for white middle-class femininity. Both Desmond and Koritz challenge the canonization of St. Denis and Allan as universally feminist role models within dance history by politicizing the fact that both choreographers capitalized on images of subjugated "Oriental" women. Koritz goes so far as to consider how white British women played dual roles as oppressors and oppressed in the interplay between Orientalism, nationalism, colonialism, and sexism.

> The similarity between Orientalism and Femininity as ideological constructs placed a Western woman performing the East in a complex position. In order to retain the privileges of her ethnicity, she cannot be too closely identified with the Orientalised subject peoples of the British Empire. At the same time, the Oriental has already been defined as "feminine" in relation to the "masculine" colonial power. Allan cannot, in this symbolic system, inhabit the privileged ground of the "masculine" West, but she can avoid the "bad" femininity of the Oriental woman. She (or her reviewers) can manipulate the distinction between a "good" and a "bad" femininity in order to position her performances on the positive side of a symbolic system that denies women full subjecthood in any case.[15]

If the Oriental represents the femininity that white women can borrow while avoiding its negative connotations through racial differences, what is the fate of the dancing Asian female body that is not allowed the separation between performances of gender and those of race and national identity? *Radha* and *Salome* demonstrate the extent to which the Asian or Asian American body can be voided of its physicality and abstracted into a collection of symbols. The problem faced by Asian American choreographers (particularly women) becomes twofold. St. Denis and Allan capitalize on the tensions between the white body and the sensuality of the Oriental dancing girl, but the Asian female body offers no such visual reminder that she is in fact performing. Since the dancing Asian female body has been reified by early modern dance as that of the morally suspect Oriental dancing girl, she cannot escape the trope through visual incongruity as white women can. The Asian female dancing body is authentically Oriental unless she directs the viewer to see otherwise.

Orientalism affects how modernity in twentieth-century U.S. culture is historicized as aesthetic innovation. After a century of cumulative cultural appropriations, each particular instance of obvious appropriation is cordoned off as an isolated artistic moment. The historical trajectory of Orientalism in U.S. "art dance" is characterized as a singular phenomenon occurring primarily in the quaintness of early-twentieth-century political innocence. Although Ruth St. Denis's Orientalist choreographies offer an unambiguous moment in Western dance history that reveals how Asian aesthetics are inextricable from contemporary U.S. culture, "Asian aesthetics" as a category continues to be considered foreign or opposite to "Western culture and values."[16] Asian American choreographers working in modern and postmodern dance vocabularies continually find themselves and their work at odds with an Orientalist discourse invested in explaining Asian American artistic innovation through the reinscription of an East-West binary.

In order to understand this discrepancy, it is necessary to take a closer look at how U.S. dance history (de)racializes and depoliticizes aesthetics. To maintain a genealogical narrative of U.S. cultural and artistic progress without admitting inextricable Asian influences, U.S. dance history uses feminist narratives that equate white female genius with the innovation of modern aesthetics. The story of American modern dance retold over and again begins with Isadora Duncan, Ruth St. Denis, Martha Graham, and Doris Humphrey, whose fierce individualism and limitless creativity defined the parameters of the American spirit of modern dance. Their oft-repeated biographies are reiterated in such a way that the language used to describe these choreographers and their careers draws on the rhetoric of the American frontier and its encounters with the other.

For those of us who believe ourselves to be enlightened consumers of avant-garde Western dance traditions, Ruth St. Denis is our foremother. She is our feminist heroine who, like Isadora Duncan, refused the corset, carved out a space for woman-the-artist, and embraced popular culture in a society ready to punish white, middle-class women for excess and independence. St. Denis's legacy has come to symbolize liberation for female dancers, even though her Orientalist practices create a hermetically sealed trap for *actual* Asian women. After St. Denis, the dancing Asian body can only be the authentic source to be drawn from directly, or viewed as the fragmented and hybridized body eternally unable to reconcile a whole self. In the latter case, it is an inauthentic and polluted body unable to be the *source* of accurate or reliable cultural knowledge (Trinh, 1989).

Suzanne Shelton (1981), Jane Desmond (1991), and Sally Banes (1998) have situated St. Denis's Oriental choreographies within a U.S. cultural context that aligns St. Denis's work conceptually with European Orientalism rather than with the specificities of U.S. Orientalism. St. Denis's encounter with the display of "natives" in their "authentic" settings at the 1901 World's Fair in Paris, her viewing of David Belasco's 1900 U.S. production of *Madame Butterfly*, and her legendary 1904 sighting of the Egyptian Deities–brand cigarette advertisement have been mythologized as three key historical moments that inspired St. Denis's career.[17] These exotic encounters can be understood through a theoretical reading of Said's mapping of European Orientalism; however, situating St. Denis within U.S. Orientalism offers a different narrative: one that demonstrates how the construction of Oriental bodies at the turn of the twentieth century continues to plague contemporary Asian American subjects a century later.

St. Denis's choreographic ingenuity is attributed to her collapse of high- and low- art dance vocabularies done in the service of producing a new dance and female persona that was at once spiritual, sensual, feminine, and feminist. The standard narrative of St. Denis's Orientalism characterizes Orientalism as the point of access for St. Denis to redefine U.S. womanhood against the strictures of white Victorian femininity. Missing from this history is a discussion of how St. Denis also collapsed the popular and academic Orientalisms that produced and sustained anti-Asian immigrant legislation in the United States well in to the second half of the twentieth century. Historians attempting to reconcile St. Denis's unmistakably Oriental aesthetic within U.S. nationalist narratives often set St. Denis's constructed representations of racial otherness apart from popular culture and align her appropriation with a depoliticized academic Orientalism. In her critique of Desmond, Sally Banes argues,

> Although Kendall sees orientalism as style, St. Denis, in the Emersonian tradition, saw it as an alternative moral system. Thus her eclectic, cross-cultural borrowing must be seen in a more complex way, historically situated, than facile charges of cultural appropriation can supply. In a way, American national identity was constructed

through imagining the other, bypassing Europe. Somehow the appropriation of otherness was transformed, in the rhetoric of the times, into constituting a quintessentially American quality.[18]

There is a magical quality to the transformative moment marked in the "somehow." That optimistic sense of wonder obscures the role Orientalism played in the United States as the method used in the regulation of Asian bodies—in particular, Asian labor in a post-emancipation United States.

By the 1906 premiere of St. Denis's *Radha*, the United States had already implemented a series of anti-Asian immigration laws in response to the growing presence of Asian laborers. Anti-Asian immigration laws never ended the importation of Asian labor since the government recognized employers' needs for a source of cheap labor once slavery was abolished. U.S. employers sought out Asian bodies to replace chattel slavery. Robert Lee argues that the Free Soil and Free Labor movement found strongest support in New England after the emancipation of slaves from the region in 1780, as a way of erasing the region's history as a slaveholding society. By the 1840s and '50s, colonization replaced abolition as the new focus of progressive social politics. Ralph Waldo Emerson, to whom St. Denis is often compared, was an enthusiastic supporter of repatriating slaves to Africa in order to build a U.S. society that was not only free of slavery but free of black bodies. Debates over the legal status of Free Soil states, such as California, were driven by the desire to contain the spread of African American populations. Importing Asian labor provided an ideal solution. Using lessons learned in the wake of slavery, the U.S. government did not categorize Asian laborers as "slaves." Instead, they were regulated through restrictive immigration and naturalization laws based on race. By barring Asians from being naturalized, the U.S. government could import Asian labor as needed without having to address the embarrassing question of slavery and its relationship to citizenship. The U.S. government had therefore, even prior to their arrival, legislated the ability to physically remove Asian immigrant populations from U.S. borders.

In racializing immigrant populations, the U.S. government was able to justify the first race-based immigration laws, beginning in 1882 with the Chinese Exclusion Act. By 1924, the state attempted to end all Asian immigration to the United States as California farmers turned their attention toward Mexico as their main source of labor.[19] Supporters of Asian labor argued for the economic necessity of Asian and Mexican laborers to fulfill the United States' Manifest Destiny. To maintain a racialized labor pool, the discourse of Orientalism provided the necessary framework in which to justify anti-Asian legislation. Orientalist discourse institutionalized the still-current belief that Asian cultural beliefs are fundamentally incompatible with the fabric of U.S. social infrastructures. Beginning with the Chinese, Asian immigrants were accused of moral depravity in the form of prostitution and homosexuality.[20]

Anti-Asian rhetoric, coupled with anti-Asian immigration laws, succeeded in making invisible the Asian American subject. When I teach, I am still at a loss when it comes time to give my lecture on Ruth St. Denis. Historically, St. Denis's 1906 *Radha* has always been remembered as a solo, even though photographs documenting the performance show a number of Indian men performing on stage with St. Denis. Even if historians do acknowledge the physical presence of these men, the men's Indian-ness renders St. Denis "authentic" and powerful while, at the same time, the men are desexualized and made inconsequential.

Banes's description of the choreography includes the fact that St. Denis as Radha performed with an entourage of "priests" who were on stage with her and part of her "act." Banes's feminist reading of *Radha* lies in the interpretation that Radha, though in the presence of men, is not dancing for the visual or sexual pleasure of men. Integral to this argument is the observation that St. Denis does not interact with the men on stage. Shelton identifies St. Denis's entourage of "Hindus" as "colored men."

As her fame and fee increased, Ruth had problems with her company of Indians. One of her stage attendants, Mahomet Ismail, sued her on the grounds that he had invented her dances, but his suit was dismissed in court. Those Hindus who remained loyal to St. Denis were vegetarians who kept their own kind of kosher on tour. They refused to eat food they considered unclean, and when their special food hampers accidentally were left behind in Chicago, they fasted for thirty-six hours on the way to Boston. They were labeled "colored" in Jim Crow America. In 1915 Ruth told a reporter that she did not dare book this early company south of the Mason Dixon line because of the overt hostility of railway and streetcar conductors. Even in the North the Hindus could not stay at the same hotels as St. Denis or travel in her train compartment.[21]

This is the extent to which St. Denis's Indian company members are acknowledged. Obviously, American antimiscegenation laws would foreclose any suggestions of a love affair between a "colored" man and a white woman. Late-nineteenth-century and early-twentieth-century narratives of interracial love between white men and "Oriental" women always ended in tragedy. The "beauty" of such stories is most often at the expense of the Oriental woman, who must commit suicide in order to be heroic. In this way, the love story remains intact, while failure of miscegenation can be moralized through the death of the Oriental woman.

The reading of St. Denis's aloofness toward the priests on stage also reinforces the way in which Asian men are feminized and asexualized. "Real" Indian men on stage cannot possibly consume St. Denis's dancing body given their position within the performance. The men merely provide an authentic backdrop for Denis's claims to transcendence. Not only are the Indian men racialized as "colored," but they are also Orientalized. Like black bodies, they pose the threat of racial pollution; but, like Chinese bodies, they also pose a social threat by subverting normative white heterosexual masculinity. Anti-Asian immigration laws limited the number of women who could enter the country, thus creating a transient Asian bachelor society. Since antimiscegenation laws forbade the marriage of "colored" men to white women, there was little social or legal possibility for Asian men to establish a nuclear family in the United States.

Opponents of Asian immigration used the results of this logic to claim that Asian populations in the United States threatened American social infrastructures because they did not live within a nuclear family structure. In the late nineteenth century, American immigration laws also barred Chinese women from entering the United States, creating a predominantly male Chinese society on American soil. This was done in order to discourage the growth of a domestic Chinese American population. The exclusion of Chinese immigrants was then justified by accusations that immigrant Chinese men were sexual deviants because they did not engage in normative heterosexual relationships in the form of nuclear family structures. They were accused of frequenting imported Chinese prostitutes, engaging in homosexual behavior, and abstaining from sex altogether. All of these activities constituted an affront to American mores. This legislated desexualization of Asian men has continued to inform popular representations of Asian masculinity. While U.S. immigration law removed Asian men from their families, effectively desexualizing them, Orientalist ideology feminized them.

Broadly, Orientalism politically feminizes the East; in particular, the Indian men on stage with St. Denis are doubly feminized as spiritual authentics. St. Denis managed to neutralize a sexualized dancing female body through her affinity with Asian spirituality. The Indian men who appeared with her on stage provided the cultural and racial authentication that St. Denis needed in order to distinguish her repertoire from that of the scandalous exotic dances (such as the hootchie cootchie) that were popular in vaudeville and in dime museums where St. Denis began her career. Dance historians have always been careful to distinguish St. Denis's interpretations of the East from attempts at ethnographic accuracy. This distinction provides more reason to consider the theatrical function of St. Denis's cast of Indian men. Historically speaking, her Orientalism has been reconciled through the disclaimer that she never intended to depict authentic Indian dance; however, the presence of Indian men on her stage provided her audience with authenticity via her affinity with authentic-looking bodies. There is contradiction in a dance history that wants to see St. Denis's performance of the Orient as an individual act that speaks to modernist notions of self-expression, while her cast of Indian men provided the evidence to support unspoken but visually evident claims to authenticity.

If St. Denis was able to use gauzy images of sensuality as a way to liberate the Victorian female body and play at the edge of sensuality and spirituality in her Orientalist choreographies, her Asian female counterparts were not as lucky. Chinese women were dehumanized as sexual commodities and reduced to potential orifices.[22] St. Denis's participation in Belasco's production of *Madame Butterfly* served as a template of Puccini's now-classic opera, which became the stereotypical trope that has followed Asian American women well into the twenty-first century. Madame Butterfly as child-bride and geisha has been recycled for over a century to instill the fantasy that institutionalized military prostitution, mail-order brides, and the Asian sex tourism industry should be viewed as models of normative Asian female sexuality (Marchetti, 1993; Hamamoto, 1994; Yamamoto, 1999; Kurahashi, 1999; and Moy, 1993).

The 1960s and '70s would mark another era when Eastern aesthetics would reemerge at defining moments in U.S. dance history. Characterized as a response to the social turmoil cause by the Vietnam War and the civil rights movement, the work of Merce Cunningham, Steve Paxton, and other post-modern choreographers is credited with revolutionizing U.S. modern dance by deconstructing choreographic structures and inventing new movement techniques using the *I Ching,* Zen Buddhism, aikido, and tai chi (Banes, 1983; Novack, 1990). The latter half of the twentieth century would see the emergence of a new Oriental body created in tandem with a continuous string of race wars fought in Asia (World War II, the Korean War, and the Vietnam War) and a major shift in immigration law.[23] The elimination of the National Origins Quota in 1965 changed U.S. immigration patterns and opened U.S. borders to an influx of Asian immigrants who met preferences for college-educated, white-collar professionals. These new immigrants, along with Japanese Americans rebuilding their lives after their internment during World War II, form the backbone of the model-minority stereotype. The model minority, complemented by "gooks" (murderous Vietcong) and "me so horny" prostitutes (formerly, bejeweled evil warlords and deflowered geishas), provides the domestic backdrop against which white middle-class men and women reasserted the innovative supremacy of (white) U.S. postmodern dancers. Postmodern dance history embraces high modernist ideals, including movement for the sake of movement, dances about choreography, and the selective borrowing of the other. Such a history closes itself off to the complexities of U.S. Orientalism.

The invisibility of Orientalism in American modern and postmodern dance history poses a problem for Asian American choreographers. Asian Americans are not viewed as abstract bodies engaging in artistic experiments. Instead, they are seen through an Orientalist double vision in which their bodily Asian-ness must remain distanced from the modern and postmodern dance vocabularies they are using. American dance aesthetics must be wholly Westernized in order to maintain a binary between the West as continuous renewal and the East as a repository of traditional source material. While white Western choreographers can mask appropriation through accounts of inspiration, Asian American performance aesthetics are stereotyped as attempts to fuse or blend incompatible Eastern and Western sensibilities. The fact that American modern and postmodern dance are *already* Asian American is denied, which leads to an Orientalist reading of Asian American choreography as a reflection of deeply rooted, biological, racial truths. In 1979, a reviewer described the work of the Asian New Dance Coalition in these terms:

> Every so often a group of choreographers joins forces. Usually it is for economic reasons or to relieve the individual artists of the responsibility of an entire program. Reynaldo Alejandro, Saeko Ichinohe, Sun Ock Lee, and Eleanor S. Yung seem to have come together for a deeper reason. One might dare to call it spiritual. . . . [H]ow would one know, other than through subject matter, that the next three works were by Oriental choreographers? It was apparent in the concentration. All had great inner stillness.[24]

Asian American choreographers are not considered to be continuing an American tradition of using spirituality to revitalize the American dance scene. Moreover, "Oriental" dancing bodies are characterized as both spiritual and unmoving. The reviewer can only see Asian bodies through the stereotype of the silent, bodiless model minority.

The work of Asian American choreographer Eleanor Yung was continually reviewed as an attempt to bridge her eternally hyphenated self. This conflict is attributed to fundamental cultural differences that are found in the dance form itself. "Traditional" movement vocabulary provides the "authentic" material, while modern and postmodern dance provide the framework for innovation. In other words, Yung can remain inherently Asian in a new context. In a review titled "Asian Balm," Bill Moore describes Yung's work as drawn from

> ageless mysteries of ancient Asian cultures. . . . Yung's dances, in fact, seem to be a strange combination of ancient Chinese and Asian movements with a lucidly clear modern dance technique. . . . The juxtaposition of the more than 2,000-year-old [*sic*] movements with the contemporary technique can, at times, be mindboggling for someone who can follow the separate threads.[25]

Another reviewer reduces Asian-ness to the role of ritual, while identifying austerity as a uniquely modern innovation.

> Although the fusion of Eastern ritual and the spare aesthetics of modern movement call for a low-keyed control and austereness, somehow an element of color and excitement must surface. . . . Though promising, Ms. Yung's pieces did not provide a fresh look at what two disparate traditions could offer. . . . It was not until the program's final piece, "Passage," was performed that Ms. Yung's ideas came into their own. A 1979 signature piece, it is a graceful amalgam of Asian ritual and modern movement. It had the most Asian look of all the dances, with kimono-clad dancers performing a graceful line of gestures and steps diagonally across the stage.[26]

Despite the fact that austerity and minimalism have been attributed to Asian aesthetic influence in modern and postmodern dance, the reviewers insist on maintaining that the two traditions are diametrically opposed. Rosemary Newton writes this about Saeko Ichinohe:

> Her work is a blend of her traditional Japanese background with the virtuosic technique of her Western dance training. It is hard to pin down Saeko's style because she choreographs both very traditionally Japanese pieces such as "Hitofude-Gaki (Drawing with one stroke)," a wonderfully sad solo for which she won the St. Denis award last year, as well as more American all-out dancing pieces such as "Asa no Uta (Ballad of morning)" with a lot in between. But in every piece one can discern the artistic bridge she is forming between her Japanese past and her more American present.[27]

"All-out dancing" is considered a bodily performance of American-ness, while Japanese-ness is a combination of national origins and a reference to a dance that seems to suggest minimalism. Japan functions as tradition, which is diametrically opposed to Ichinohe's Juilliard dance education. Can the same be said for postmodern appropriations of Buddhism, Taoism, yoga, or whatever Asian philosophy is in vogue? There are no contradictions between aesthetics and race as national identity when white postmodernists are discussed. No one suspects Merce Cunningham, Robert Dunn, Anna Halprin, or Steve Paxton of exploring a national identity that is not wholly and universally American.

Conclusion

After revisiting Sue Li-Jue's *The Nature of Nature*, I would say that I agree with Belmar's comments that the monologue text needed more work and the choreography relied a little too heavily on "leggy" modern dance vocabulary, but the *grand battements* and *arabesques* were always preceded or followed by double barrel turns, quirky torso releases, rolls, dives, and/or moments of stillness. In other words, Li-Jue looks to modern dance vocabularies in order to find a way in which to present on stage a spectacle of Asian female bodies that are strong and athletic, and that articulate agency enacted through bodily interpretation of the movement generated from an ethos of aesthetic abstractions. An Asian Americanist reading of the work tries to make visible the Asian aesthetic that is already imbedded in the history of modern dance itself, an aesthetic that becomes a form of politics. This complex negotiation is hard to see when the dancers' bodies are always already racially marked, and narrativized before they start to move.

Rethinking postmodern dance's and contact improvisation's parodoxical practices of Orientalism and disavowal of Asian bodies leads into another set of concerns. I find a similarity between the mythology of contact improvisation's portrayal as a democratic dance form and the mythology of Asian American performance art as an expansion of democratic representation. Sociologically speaking, the idea that Asian American performance exists adds to the multicultural fantasy that the United States has become a more tolerant and inclusive place. Asian American performance art as the last frontier of artistic and political radicalism is "proof" that Asian Americans, too, can participate on the cutting edge of sociological inclusion in the United States. The "inclusion" of Asian American performance by way of "being present"—though not necessarily included—functions as demographic evidence that multiculturalism is working to include Asian Americans.

Asian American performance artists use the principles of postmodern dance and contact improvisation within their work *because* the techniques are considered democratic and inclusive. But, as with literature and film, performance within the Asian American community continues to function as ethnic representation. Asian American performance has not been able to escape the realm of "community theater," while white postmodern dance and contact improvisation have managed to claim a politics of community practice while at the same time becoming artistically universalized techniques.

The idea that Asian American performance is a consciousness-raising forum that inspires other Asian Americans to pursue performance art as a career is not unlike the appeal of contact improvisation. Asian American performance does take on the task of presenting performance to communities who otherwise feel excluded from mainstream art programming. Like postmodern dance and its legacy of improvisation, Asian American performance has also been mythologized as a politically liberating and artistically radical genre within the genealogy of artistic discourse, while continuing to serve as an entertaining diversion in the realm of "serious politics." The idealized concept of "process over product" can be heard in both socio-artistic circles.

The affinity between Asian American performance and the democratic ideals of postmodern dance practices is also a double-edged sword. Using the rhetoric of democracy does affect how and where Asian American performance is produced. The idea that Asian American performance should both draw from the community and be available to a community generates the perception that the performance should be staged under less-than-ideal circumstances because of social responsibility and not necessarily by artistic choice. Certainly site-specific or public arts projects demonstrate the value placed on reflecting and creating community, but this is a separate issue from situations in which Asian American performance artists are pressured to make their work available despite inappropriate and/or inadequate technical support.

What I have attempted to outline in this chapter are the disciplinary stakes of situating dance in Asian American studies and Asian American studies within dance. To return to Sue Li-Jue's *Facing East* as an example: it would be easy locate her work as demonstrating the complexity of Asian American culture because of how she consciously names her moves between the overtly political and the overtly aesthetic, but she ultimately fails to satisfy critics who want to hear Asian American political wit and critics who want to see formal experimentation. It is this moment of dissatisfaction from both ends that reveals failed moments within the interdisciplinary project and provides a window into the stakes for claiming an Asian American dance studies.

2

CLUB O' NOODLES'S
LAUGHTER FROM THE CHILDREN OF WAR

Imagine driving down Interstate 10, exiting at Cloverfield, merging into
the left turn lane, and in the few seconds right after the green light turns
red, you turn onto Olympic Boulevard. You made it. Now imagine turn-
ing right on 18th, where you slowly cruise up and down the street looking
for a parking space. You get out of the car, walk up to the ticket counter
inside an inconspicuous building, and buy your $12 ticket. Imagine
standing in the foyer noticing the names of people painted on the floor,
realizing suddenly that you are in a gallery, that the names on the floor
represent people who have died of AIDS, that the black-and-white photo-
graphs displayed on the wall depict two men in an embrace and a close-up
shot of a penis. Imagine that you notice those waiting with you are
families, families with children, Vietnamese families with children. Sud-
denly you realize that this is the first time that you have seen Asian
families in a space coded as queer.

In bringing a Vietnamese American audience into a "queer" space, Club O'
Noodles accomplished the more difficult task of countering multicultural
programming practices that assume unidirectional movement of knowledge,
whereby lessons on Vietnamese American culture and history are delivered
to a white audience. Within this model of multiculturalism, which Lisa
Lowe calls "aestheticized multiculturalism," the body of a racialized subject
represents a vessel of preserved ethnic identity, while the white subject represents a homogenized mainstream identity that becomes "aware" without
risking its social standing as the mainstream referent.[1] Narratives of assimilation usually presuppose the movement from margins to the mainstream,
but, in this case, the contact between the Vietnamese family-as-community

(coded as heteronormative and socially conservative) and Highways Performance Space (coded as white, queer, and liberal) is altogether another story. When these entities are placed within the same space, it is unclear which category of other is more other, thus providing an example of how visible intersections of race, gender, sexuality, and class are sometimes met with silence. Is it effective for young children to view large photographs of genitalia? The scheduled performance event operates as an interlocutor between these two constituencies; part of the challenge of writing about Club O' Noodles's work is analyzing it from both an aesthetic and a social perspective without collapsing or ignoring the interdependence of the two.

I first saw *Laughter from the Children of War* (1995) in the winter of 1995, and my field notes indicate that I was struck by the presence of a largely Vietnamese audience in a queer space. But it was the actual performance itself that inspired this project. Memories of laughing out loud and fighting back tears while sitting in the audience motivate this chapter, as I present an account of what happened once the house lights dimmed, the performance began, and the audience and the space disappeared. This close reading of *Laughter from the Children of War* follows the structure of the piece from beginning to end in an effort both to provide the reader with a sense of how the work is structured and to represent as much as possible what it looked like on stage. Descriptions are always interpretive, and it is not my intention to propose the possibility of fully capturing live performance in writing. Thick description (Geertz, 1973) in this case is (1) an analysis of the themes presented in the work as they are revealed by the choreographic structure of the piece, and (2) a way to communicate in writing the non-text-based elements of multidisciplinary performances that incorporate movement, text, and song.[2] Club O' Noodles's choreographic use of the transition between scenes (how they juxtapose the beginnings and endings of individual scenes) operates as an important aesthetic device in the disruption of fixed meanings and identities within individual scenes. Stylistically, Club O' Noodles uses a series of non sequiturs to create a nonlinear narrative that generates humor, irony, and satire.

Following the assumption that the performers are themselves in the process of theorizing issues of representation, stereotype, and identity in the execution of the piece, my descriptive analysis follows the sequence of the performance. This writing strategy is different from choosing to highlight excerpts from *Laughter* as illustrative examples of a given theme. This does not mean that I am not interested in discussing the social and political issues addressed in the performances, but my intention is to reveal (1) how the performance is a self-representation in time and space and (2) how the performers reveal content through form.

Dance scholars grapple with the challenge of translating movement into writing. On a basic level, how does one describe a *pas de bourrée* without assuming that everyone knows what that means? How to do it without sounding like a how-to dance manual? Add to this a situation in which the music, text, and set are important narrative components. Within Asian American performance history, as noted by Josephine Lee (1997), the documentation of Asian American performance history occurs primarily through the publication of a playscript. But this kind of documentation suggests that the texts are written before they are performed. Different from anthologies of playscripts, *Tokens?*(A. Eng, 1999) includes a number of multidisciplinary performance projects—including choreography, text, music, installations— translated from live performance into scripted text for the purpose of record keeping. Performances with this text-based component do lend themselves to direct translation, but there is a risk of collapsing all genres of performance into one representative model. In "No Menus Please (Three Delivery Guys Riding in a Circle on Tricycles)," a stage direction included after the fourth monologue reads "Choreographed cycling, collision and slow motion falls" (*Tokens?* 306). As a reader, I would imagine that the moment when the performers collapse is as important, if not more important, than the rest of the script.

How is it possible to account for what the body is doing and revealing on stage? If a discursive move toward aesthetics can be made such that critique of Asian American cultural production can move away from "the sociology of the Asian American experience" and toward an aesthetic study of Asian American performance (Xing 44), then critics and scholars alike *must* find languages and methodologies to account for the choreographic structure of performance work. The following analysis of *Laughter from the Children of War* examines how choreographic choices and movement vocabulary drive the narrative of each performance to make evident how movement and text comment on each other in order to create multiple meanings indiscernible from written text alone. This is a move toward recognizing the kinetic execution of the "choreography of identity" as a deliberation that is different from purely linguistic performances of identity.

Reading *Laughter*

Between 1995 and 1999, Club O' Noodles toured *Laughter from the Children of War* across the United States as a work-in-progress representing the experience of Vietnamese immigration in Southern California. Developed by Hung Nguyen and Nobuko Miyamoto, *Laughter* is based on a series of autobiographical and fictional stories accumulated over a two-year period of rehearsals and performance workshops. Club O' Noodles implements postmodern choreographic strategies to envision a collective, yet historically specific, portrayal of Vietnamese American subjectivities. In combining text, movement, and music, the ensemble composes an immigrant body that challenges Orientalist representations of Asian bodies and broaches topics considered taboo by the Vietnamese American community.[3]

Issues such as welfare, sexuality, and the experience of the boat people are discussed publicly on stage. The latter is a crucial element in the performance, since a large majority of the performers were born in the late 1960s and early 1970s and came to the United States during the second wave of Vietnamese immigration. Many of the members were boat children who experienced life in refugee camps in Thailand, Malaysia, and the United States. Club O' Noodles does not consider *Laughter* an attempt to represent a universal experience, valid for all Vietnamese immigrants, but rather makes salient notions of community and the diversity within the community. It destabilizes the image of a homogeneous diasporic community tied by a common country of origin, and in its place presents a multilingual narrative referencing mass media, popular culture, English as a second language, and Vietnamese as a "forgotten" language.

The characters portrayed in *Laughter* are based on the company members' perception of themselves and other Vietnamese immigrants in their own extended families, neighborhoods, and schools.[4] These perceptions include their internalized stereotypes of who and what a Vietnamese immigrant is. The company relies on potentially dangerous reiterations of stereotypes to transform stock characters into individuals, thus challenging their audiences' desire to see both the disintegration and the reappearance of stereotype. Characters matching stereotypical expectations push the limits of what is considered funny versus what is true. *Laughter* does not disavow the representation of the Vietnamese immigrant, but resignifies stereotypical images by re-presenting real and imagined episodes of Vietnamese immigrant life. The performers' bodies "flesh out" and disturb the superficial nature of stereotypes by providing glimpses of self-prescribed stereotypes, counterstereotypes, and childhood memories cross-referenced through fragmented scenes that simultaneously conflict and support one another.

Composed of twenty independent scenes, the most extensive version of *Laughter* can be up to two hours long, featuring both recurring and non-recurring characters played by a rotating cast. The fluid terms of staging and casting affect the overall look of the work. For the sake of consistency, my analysis is based on a set of notes I took during a performance at the Dance Studio Theater at the University of California, Riverside, on May 16, 1996. Those notes were supplemented by repeated viewings of the video recording. Since I have seen multiple versions of the performance in different venues with different cast members, I will take the liberty of writing about scenes or choreographic choices that did not necessarily occur in the performance at UC Riverside, but were repeatedly included in later productions. In doing so, my intention is to gain insights into what the performers as a collective consider to be the most relevant aspects of *Laughter*.

The Scenes

For the purposes of this essay, I will describe and analyze six scenes that the performers considered the most important or representative of the work. Given that the performers presented shorter versions of *Laughter* (as short as forty-five minutes), certain scenes were consistently selected to represent the main body of the work. These scenes differ dramatically from each other both aesthetically and thematically. For example, a full-length *Laughter* includes four different "Family Scenes," but only one or two of them are considered core, defining scenes, while the others are elaborations deemed expendable in shortened versions of the performance. Combinations of specific sequences recur, creating a balanced presentation of dialogue, music, singing, and movement. Two scenes that depend heavily on dialogue are never performed one after another. Instead, scenes with more emphasis on movement and/or music precede or follow a monologue or a dialogue. The same goes for energy and emotional content: an upbeat or humorous scene always follows or precedes one that is somber or quiet. Choreographically, the juxtaposition of contrasts presents a wide range of approaches and responses to the issues brought forth in the performance.[5]

"FAIRY TALES"

The performance begins with a voiceover text that at first sounds like a Disneyfied version of a children's fairytale. A man's soothing voice narrates over the sound of slow-paced traditional Vietnamese stringed instruments:

> Once upon a time, not too long ago, in a land not too far away, there lived a Dragon Prince and a Fairy Princess. They met, fell in love, and eventually bred one hundred eggs that become lots of children.[6]

Initially, the performance looks and sounds like an exotic Asian fairy tale about the genesis of the Vietnamese people, complete with ancient dragons and princesses. After this momentary seduction, the tale moves from a fictive past into recent history. The entire stage is covered with mounds of newspaper and lit with blue light that creates dark shadows between the mounds.

The scene is reminiscent of a cloudy mountaintop, a forlorn landscape, or a heap of trash. A weblike curtain made of "strings" of newspaper hangs from ceiling to floor across the back of the stage. The mounds of newspaper begin to rustle and move ever so slightly, giving away the secret that bodies are hidden under the piles of newspaper. The narration continues; and what began as a mythic fairy tale turns quickly into a story of domestic strife and a parable for the civil war in Vietnam. The narrator's languid voice remains the same, heightening the performance's dark sense of humor as the content of the story transitions from fairy tale to allegorical soap opera.

> Then one day, like a typical dysfunctional family, the Prince and Princess decided to get a divorce. And it was a nasty divorce at that. At first, the Princess took some children to the Northern mountain, and the rest went to the Southern sea with their father. Like any other divorce, they needed lawyers to advise them on how to fight for their rights. So the Prince and Princess hired world famous

lawyers to defend them. Because both the lawyers argued so well, the fight went on for over thirty years.

At this point, the ten bodies concealed underneath the newspapers begin to "hatch" and a hand, elbow, or foot slowly emerges from each giant newspaper bubble. The sound of tearing newspaper accompanies the sight of disembodied limbs growing out of the ground. Arms, fingers, and legs emerge twisted. Heads and trunks are the last body parts the audience sees.

The humor of the "dysfunctional family" is layered against the action of the performers as they lie on the floor contracted in fetal positions, then writhe through a series of awkward shapes as they move into standing positions. Their writhing bodies indicate both birth and death as they stir with and against the text. Our expectations of a traditional myth are shattered when the tale references American pop psychology—the stuff of afternoon talk shows—and, finally, civil war. The term "dysfunctional family" situates the performers within a milieu familiar with an American culture that gives a clinical name to the breaking apart of families. The irony is even more effective when the voiceover uses "dysfunctional family" both to reference the destruction of nation and to challenge stereotypes of the model-minority Asian American family structure.

The performers' bodies are all of a sudden inhabiting multiple geographic locations as the text continues to spiral toward a darker reality, told in the language of U.S. corporate culture.

They fought and fought and fought until both the Prince and Princess had no money left. So the lawyers quit. Now that all the blood-slinging, bomb-dropping, and name-calling had settled, the Prince and Princess realized that some of their children had run away from home.

Finally reaching a full standing position, the performers in slow motion, pumping their arms back and forth, appear to sprint across the stage. Dressed in variations on black T-shirts and denim jeans, the cast look like a group of teenage friends as they move across the diagonals of the stage. Eventually, they traverse and cover the entire stage and begin to sing a traditional Vietnamese lullaby.

This kind of linguistic switch between English text and Vietnamese lyrics continues throughout the bilingual performance without the aid of translation. Although it is not always necessary to understand Vietnamese in order to follow the performance, many of the jokes are told in Vietnamese and serve as a marker for monitoring who in the audience is or is not included as Vietnamese American and Asian American. The laughter generated by the in-jokes provides an aural map as to where the Vietnamese-speakers sit in the darkened theater.

The performers continue to sing in Vietnamese without pause when the sound of rap music fades in. Eventually, one of the men stumbles to center stage, stops singing, and looks around in confusion as 2 Live Crew's "Naughty by Nature" increases in volume. He takes out a pair of sunglasses hidden in the waistband of his pants, slips the sunglasses on, and begins a series of pelvic thrusts and shoulder rolls. He moves toward the audience and cheers. Eventually the other performers notice the soloist's change in movement dynamics, and, one at a time, stop both their sprinting and singing. One by one, the performers pull out sunglasses and tentatively join the soloist's movement sequence until everyone has mastered the hip-hop routine and the entire ensemble is moving in unison.

The sight of ten Asian bodies wearing sunglasses on a dark stage and executing an exaggerated hip-hop routine while screaming in ecstasy renders laughter and cheering from the audience. Eventually the group falls out of unison as members of the audience are invited on stage to join in what suddenly becomes a dance party. The performers gyrate and bounce in groups of two and three, performing their own individual styles of movement in time with the rap song. Moving in close proximity to one another, the dancers gesture for the audience to notice their cool moves. One by one the dancers try to upstage each other and hold center stage, until they start turning violent against one another.

"Freaking" turns into pushing, punching, and jumping on top of one another. They shred and throw newspaper into the air, holler at one another, and a body is suddenly lifted and propelled through space in a swirl of trash. The heightened state of frenzy slowly dies down, as individuals "drop dead" one or two at a time, until no one is left standing. Throughout this time, the audience members who were brought on stage are never led off stage or given any direction as the fight escalates. They are most often left on their own to digest the sudden turn in events and to find their way back to their seats when they discover that they no longer belong on stage. A moment of silence follows and the performers resume singing their lullaby again, but this time it is barely audible.

Through simple juxtapositions of energy qualities within the choreographic design (the slow and fearful movement performed to the lullaby, the forceful and loose quality of the hip-hop sequence, and the direct jerking action in the fight scene), the group improvises social interactions that can be read on many different levels. The scene brings about images of assimilation, conformity, confusion, and violence, but it is not clear where this is taking place geographically. Chronological references are equally confusing. The hip-hop sequence evokes the process of assimilation to U.S. culture, but the ensuing violence brings the performers into the same positions on stage where they began.

What does the violence refer to? The violence of war, the psychic violence of assimilation, or the impossibility of assimilation? A transformation has clearly taken place as the panicked, unwitting audience members are left on stage to look around in confusion before deciding to return to their seats. The violence of the fight scene refers back to the violence of the story told in the fairy tale. The choreographed fight and the fact that everyone "dies" also generates associations with the Vietnam War tacitly referred in the fairy tale. The bodies on stage perform both the violence of the Vietnam War and the violence of alienation in America. Memories and experiences of war in Vietnam are introduced at the beginning of the performance in a temporally fragmented manner and foreground the structure of the rest of the performance.

"FAMILY SCENE #1"

Laughter is not always geographically uncertain, though it does move fluidly between the United States and Vietnam. The following scene takes place in a U.S. cultural context. It also addresses the transitional space that new immigrants must navigate. The stereotypical representation of the Asian immigrant body as the f.o.b. family in America forces the audience to engage actively in the performance by taking on subject positions in relationship to the material presented in the work.[7]

Jokes about Asian immigrants' inept bodies and behaviors seduce the audience into responding to—and making choices about how one should react to—a funny yet hurtful stereotype. Laughter functions as a gauge of the spectator's relationship to the issues brought forth by the performance. Club O' Noodles's use of humor in *Laughter* is politically acute, since "getting" the joke requires consideration of one's relationship to the content.

Laughter includes four "Family Scenes"; however, I will focus on "Family Scene #1," which ridicules the postural and linguistic inabilities of a newly arrived Asian immigrant family, because it uses the most provocative stereotypes. I will analyze this scene in two sections. The first, "We always stick together," looks at how the immigrant body functions as a source of social embarrassment. The second—"Who is laughing at the F.O.B.?"—is a close examination of the tricks involved in taking apart a stereotype without dismantling the person. I also attempt to cast individual characteristics and actions that make up the stereotype of the F.O.B. in a positive and, hence, a different light.

"We always stick together." A cluster of five performers stand arm in arm in a circle with their backs toward each other, so that they are facing outside the circle. Together, they shuffle on stage and each performer looks around as if in amazement. The Father, played by Hung Nguyen, declares in a thick Vietnamese accent, "My family, a typical fresh-off-the-boat Vietnamese family. We always stick together. Like white on rice." He calls himself an F.O.B. before the audience gets a chance to think of him as an F.O.B., and then overperforms the stereotype. He pulls his pants up high so that the waistband sits above his waist—a reference to his "nerdiness" and unfamiliarity with "proper" American fashion—then waits a beat for the audience to notice and laugh at him. With his pants pulled too high, his Vietnamese accent, and the large family that clings to him, the character of The Father is the embodiment of the immigrant child's nightmare—The Father is the F.O.B. literally fresh off the boat, not a jet.

The phrase "We always stick together" is repeated throughout the first family scene. It plays on the idea of sticking together as a concept that requires an erasure of difference within the group in the interest of asserting an external collective difference, for protection. "We always stick together, like white on rice," The Father and his family repeat over and over again as they shuffle arm in arm. The performers poke fun at both the stereotype and the cultural alliances assumed through the words "eating rice."[8] Assumptions about eating rice are the entry/entree through which Club O' Noodles introduces larger questions of identity politics and political alliances.[9] "Sticking together, like white on rice" doesn't hold up, as the family ends up leaving The Father behind at the end of the scene.

T. Minh-ha Trinh (1989) warns against the dangers of believing that one can maintain the authenticity of the "endangered species" because preservation is impossible, as the attempt to maintain authenticity does the reverse. "Sticking together" in order to build a coalition based on "ethnic authenticity" destroys "sticking together," since it requires both a process of identification and differentiation. The process of locating authentic identity requires a group to find differences between itself and other groups of "authentics." Before a particular ethnic group can claim identity, it must stick together to establish its difference from (an)other, so as not to be confused with (an)other. In doing so, groups may be able to establish their differences from each other, but they forget that they are all (an)other fighting in the same struggle. Sticking together diverts attention away from the problem of racism and contributes to the success of a divide-and-conquer strategy.[10] The danger of falling into the trap of essential sameness is in constant tension with the trap of individualism. Both jeopardize the possibility of speaking as a viable and unified voice.

"Who is laughing at the F.O.B.*?"* When the audience members hear The Father perform his Vietnamese accent, we laugh. But what are we laughing at? Are we laughing because Asian accents are inherently funny?[11] The performer based the accent he performs on how his own father spoke English. So why is it funny to hear someone speak with an accent? This is an Asian American performance for a presumably Asian American audience, on guard whenever impersonations of Asian accents are performed for laughs. The performance plays on the audience's fears of seeing a stereotype reinforced. But it is unclear if the character of The Father is a pure stereotype or is actually based on someone's father. The Father is a reminder of the internalized Asian American fear of being embarrassed by the immigrant. Playing on the fear of encountering the F.O.B., living with one, or even being one, the performer embodies the stereotype of the F.O.B. through his voice, his posture, his expression, condensed to its purest form. Wait. Does this mean that the stereotype has some validity?[12]

Josephine Lee's 1997 analysis of David Henry Hwang's *M. Butterfly* and Philip Kan Gotanda's *Yankee Dawg You Die* argues that the Asian and Asian American characters in these two plays make visible the labor of performing Oriental stereotypes, and are thus able to "emphasize their overdetermined, literal, and pervasive manifestations" (98). Nguyen's performance of the F.O.B. father does similar work; however, the origins of the stereotypes deployed in *M. Butterfly* and *Yankee Dawg You Die* are referenced within the plays themselves as fictional media stereotypes, whereas Nguyen's performance references histories of continued migration.

Nguyen performs the immigrant's awkwardness, newness, and unfamiliarity with American culture in order to reveal how lack of familiarity is translated into a stereotype and read as deficiency. The stereotype cannot simply be disposed of: as Nguyen's performance of the immigrant father points out, The Father vacillates between the stereotype and the person. Through the stereotype, The Father draws attention to the fact that monolingual English-speaking America considers Asian-accented English unsophisticated and not fully American. Nguyen's performance demands that the audience reconsider what constitutes a stereotype, by asking what happens to a person who inhabits the characteristics that have become recognizable as the universal stereotype of Asian American–ness.

Nguyen addresses the audience directly. He tries to buy French fries as if the audience were the cashier at a fast-food restaurant. He acts overly enthusiastic. His pants are too short and his family too big. Nguyen squints at the menu as he makes the wrong word choices. Sitting in the theater, confronted with his body, the audience establishes its difference with this exaggerated performance of the Asian-immigrant stereotype. The Asian American audience faces its own fears of encountering the authentically inept immigrant body. At the same time, the audience confronts the pleasure of seeing this authentic other that allows one to establish one's distance from the image.

Nguyen consciously manipulates the role of the authentic other so central to imperialist projects of categorization, which implement stereotypes as universal indicators of difference between Us and the Other. Without costume changes, Nguyen simply shifts postures and manipulates his own clothing to indicate that he is performing The Father; so his body performs the problematic authentic other. Nguyen makes the audience aware that the stereotype is a performance by speaking in an Asian accent different from his own.

Nguyen calls himself "the F.O.B." satirically, since he did, in fact, escape from Vietnam on a boat. He performs the expectations of the F.O.B. stereotype by making a visible effort at performing non-normalized Asian immigrant—ness in order to fulfill the expectations of the stereotype. In doing so, he also calls attention to the multifaceted components of immigrant identity, flattened out to create a stereotype. At the same time, he makes clear that such complexity accounts for the reality of Vietnamese American culture. The performance risks the reiteration of the stereotype by creating a character who makes the audience uncomfortable with their complicity as spectators. Rather than accepting Nguyen's representation as true, or rejecting it as false, he challenges audience members to examine the perception of their own proximity to and difference from Nguyen's immigrant body—a body consciously engaged in a satiric performance of a stereotype.

I am laughing. The people sitting next to me are laughing. I look around; everyone in the audience is laughing. We laugh at Nguyen's body. A body searching for inflections, emphasis, dynamic variation. We laugh at his cho-reographic choices.[13] He places his punctuation, accents, variations in unex-pected places. Admit it: we don't embrace his choices as clever insights, but disdain them as deficiencies. He says to the audience, "Good morning how are you today thank you very much! Me, Su Huynh. This my family." He introduces his family, then says, "We want potato, no not French fry, potato. What? Three-fifty.... What? No food stamp ... but potato food, right?" At the end of the scene, his family eventually pulls him off stage and in unison they say, "My father knows everything. But he doesn't know English." His children dismiss him with a flick of the wrist as if swatting a fly.

Rather than rallying around his ability to shock and confuse the cashier/audience with his skill in manipulating and distorting conventions of lan-guage, we laugh at the effort. He addresses us, the audience, with his desires, and we laugh at his desires. For a moment our own identity as audience member is suspended. Are we the ones who always (however secretly, la-tently) do the laughing? Do we realize that we are laughing at someone close to us, the one we translate for? Do we laugh at ourselves reflexively or is Nguyen's bodily image a projection of the "not me?" It is uncomfortable to be confronted by our own reaction to a performance of the immigrant body. Delving into our reaction, is it one that is covertly resentful of the father's (un)skillfulness? Or do we distance ourselves by imagining for ourselves, a "sense of specialness," what Trinh describes as the division between the "I-who-have-made-it" and the "You-who-cannot-make-it"?[14]

GILLIGAN'S ISLAND AND "THE BOAT DANCE"

Audiences do not get to hold on to characters such as The Father, because once they are introduced, the performers abandon them for abstract images and concepts. Those cast in the role of the F.O.B. family do not perform as specific characters in the next scene, titled "The Boat Dance." This work is conceptualized as a choreographed movement piece based on visual images and bodily memories rather than a narrative; the performers move to center stage and strike a pose as if they were having their pictures taken for a high school yearbook. They sing the theme song from the popular 1970s television show *Gilligan's Island* and strike a new pose at the end of every refrain. The song describes the premise of the television comedy, in which a group of strangers on a weekend boat trip find themselves stranded on a tropical island after getting caught in a storm. Their poses become more expansive as they ham it up for the camera, leaning on one another, trying to upstage each other. The picture-posing sequence comes to an end and they stumble back and forth across the stage as they sing the final stanza, about the ship tossing in rough seas, closing with: "If not for the courage of the fearless crew, / the boat would be lost." In some performances, this last line is sung to the same tune but quietly, like a lullaby, as a reference back to the Vietnamese lullaby sung at the beginning of the performance. In reiterating a form, the performers create a choreographic and thematic connection between otherwise unrelated scenes.

The pace slows down; finally, everyone kneels with their foreheads touching the ground. The sound of whispering wind and flutes comes over the loudspeakers. The performers, crouched in two rows, begin rocking from side to side in unison. We hear the performers cough and moan while their arms rise and fall as if they are trying to fly. Four dancers in the back row rise to their feet, while the four dancers downstage continue rocking and crawling on the ground. The group kneeling on the floor in front reach upward until their bodies are fully extended in a high, right diagonal, momentarily suspended before diving back toward the floor. Both groups repeat this phrase in canon, creating the visual sensation that the stage is rolling and pitching back and forth. This is the only scene in the entire performance unaccompanied by spoken text. Memory here is visualized as physical movement.

To equate the experience of the boat people to the coconut-eating antics portrayed on *Gilligan's Island* borders on the absurd, the trivial, and/or the insensitive. But the absurdity of *Gilligan's Island* is part of this memory and is based on a performer's childhood recollections: "I used to watch *Gilligan's Island* when I was a kid, and it would remind me of leaving Vietnam." No spoken text accompanies "Boat Dance," as if the experience itself is silenced within both the Vietnamese American community and U.S. history at large. During rehearsals, comments such as "no one in my family talked about it [the refugee camps] after we came to America" recurred in conversation. Films like *Platoon* and *Apocalypse Now* offer larger-than-life and visually graphic depictions of the physical and psychological violence of the Vietnam War, yet it is a children's television sitcom that triggers kinetic memories of postwar survival.

Kinetic memory forms the central image of this scene, a scene without reference to a process of leaving and arriving typical of immigrant narratives. The bodies here are drifting physically and metaphorically between nations with no placeable identity; their destination is ambiguous, and, by the end of the sequence, there is no indication that they have arrived anywhere. Like Martha Graham's modernist abstractions of human emotion, "The Boat Dance" invokes a bodily expression as the primary subject of the scene. It is through the bodily performance that a historical narrative emerges.

"FROM WAR TO HOLLYWOOD IN AMERICA"

Following the boat children's stories are a series of parodic interpretations of Hollywood and Broadway productions about the Vietnam War. This pairing makes evident how the diegetic and theatrical Vietnam in films like *Rambo* and the musical *Miss Saigon* are inextricably intertwined with Vietnamese American identity. The transition into the following scene begins as the entire cast runs frantically around the stage while the sound of a helicopter buzzes overhead. The chop-chop-chop of the helicopter pauses, and the cast freezes in its tracks to sing a Vietnamese communist anthem. The sound of the helicopter starts again and the sequence is repeated three times. Each time the phrase (running then freezing in place) is repeated, the performers huddle closer together, as if the propellers of an approaching helicopter were whipping up the air. Bent forward in a stooped position, they yell at each other in Vietnamese with their faces hidden behind large, triangular straw hats. This is the classic image of Vietnamese peasants made familiar in Hollywood representations of the Vietnam War. To further play on the sentiment that U.S. soldiers could not differentiate between friend or foe, the performers sing a communist anthem that several of them had learned in Vietnam as children.

Suddenly the overture from *Miss Saigon* replaces the sound of the helicopter; a small, plastic toy helicopter descends from the ceiling on a piece of string. Looking perplexed, the cast gathers around the helicopter and a woman sings, "What is the meaning of this?" to the melody of the *Miss Saigon* overture. In unison, the performers step out of character and complain that the helicopter is only a toy. Everyone falls into a kick-line formation while one half of the cast sings, "Where's the helicopter? Where's the helicopter?" and the other half replies, "We can't do a show about Vietnam without a real helicopter! No one will pay to see the show!" H. Nguyen, now playing The Director, makes note of the ensuing chaos and calls everyone to attention: "Wait a minute guys. But this is all we can afford! Please, this is low-budget theater!"

In a doubly self-reflexive move, the performers both break the "fourth wall" of theater performance and recognize the break, in order to foreground the theatricality of the performance at hand and the theatricality of film and theater that the scene deconstructs. Citing both the media frenzy over the landing of a life-size helicopter in *Miss Saigon* and the landing of the helicopter on the Broadway stage, the appearance of the toy helicopter ties the entirety of *Miss Saigon* (the casting controversy, the employment of Asian actors, the problematic *Butterfly* narrative) to the omnipresence of helicopters in Hollywood films about the Vietnam War. Since the demographics of Vietnamese American communities are historically tied to the aftermath of the Vietnam War, Club O' Noodles's members examine their own inability to completely separate themselves as Vietnamese Americans from cultural artifacts associated with the Vietnam War. This struggle with Hollywood film and its all-encompassing representational power is manifest in the performative moment when the artists allude to their marginality not as "Vietnamese people," but as "actors."

The actor performing as The Director essentially performs as himself, while the rest of the artists perform as disgruntled actors longing for stardom but with no real chance at making it big in Hollywood or on Broadway. The actors perform as actors in their present space, alluding to the perception that Asian American actors wait it out in "alternative theater spaces," like East West Players, until their big break, contrary to the activist rhetoric of Asian American theater in which alternative theater is the theater of choice. One of the male performers runs to the front of the stage, stretches out his arms, and yells, "We don't even have enough money to pay for real actors!" A woman yells from upstage, "Hey! We could use *real* Vietnamese people!" In this exchange, the performers play with the assumptions propagated by Hollywood casting practices: according to this logic, Vietnamese people do not need to "perform" Vietnamese-ness because they are essentially Vietnamese.

Simply "looking Vietnamese" replaces the necessity for performing multidimensional characters and individuals. When one of the female performers declares, "Hey! We could use *real* Vietnamese people," she deepens the conundrum. Her commentary on the practice of casting non-Vietnamese actors in Vietnamese roles (think of *Miss Saigon*) is also a cynical statement because she suggests the use of Vietnamese people as a last resort when non-Vietnamese performers are unavailable. It becomes unclear whether she is performing as a Vietnamese or a non-Vietnamese person, given that she offered the idea of bringing Vietnamese people to perform in this show because they would do it for free. Obviously, she is a Vietnamese person performing in *Laughter,* but the performers' identities are suspended in regard to what their ethnic identities are in that moment. A final twist is introduced when one of the men responds to the suggestion: "Real Vietnamese people? I'm outta here!" and he struts off stage with several other performers following close behind. What of the difference between Vietnamese and Vietnamese American identity? Do the cast members leave in disgust because, as self-identified Vietnamese American actors or American citizens, they are no longer Vietnamese in nationality?[15]

What is so remarkable about this scene is that the audience is set up to know that all of the actors are Vietnamese and have been performing as Vietnamese characters. At this point in the performance, the performers draw attention to what they are up against in mainstream representations of Vietnamese people. The scene elicits humor because the performers are playing with the audience's ability to separate the performers' racially marked bodies from those of the characters that they are playing. Before now, the performers have been enacting diverse representations of the Vietnamese experience. At this point, they begin performing performers who are not themselves. Rather than allowing the audience to feel comfortable with the idea that they are genuine Vietnamese Americans playing Vietnamese and Vietnamese American roles, these bodies have the ability to perform as something other. Whether or not the audience is willing to see racially marked bodies perform as something other is the challenge that Club O' Noodles investigates.

Everyone starts milling around and individual performers stop in their tracks to directly address the audience. One man announces, "We can't do a show about Vietnam with no killing." The other performers turn to stab each other, then turn to the audience to ask, "No killing?!" Then the performers grab each other by the torso and mime a rape scene, and one man yells, "No raping!" They stop what they are doing, turn to the audience, and inquire, "No raping?" Placing their hands on their hips, the women gyrate their pelvises while the men lurch toward them. One of the men states, "No prostitutes," and the women turn toward the audience, asking: "No prostitutes? We're outta here." They strut off stage while the men follow, chanting, "Me so horny, me so horny, me love you long time. . . . "[16]

The formula for the Hollywood Vietnam War film is broken down into a basic list of ingredients. The scene is not so much about the Vietnam War, but the extent to which Vietnamese people, and women in particular, stand in for harbingers of violence. Death and prostitution are synonymous with Vietnamese bodies, which function as backdrops for U.S. heroics, and Vietnamese women, imagined as both rape victims and prostitutes, feature prominently in the public imagination. The prostitute in Stanley Kubrick's *Full Metal Jacket* (1987) has become the iconic Vietnamese woman made famous by delivering the oft-quoted lines, "Me so horny, me love you long time." The film, championed as a self-consciously over-the-top critique of the Vietnam War, has lost its critical edge since being reappropriated by popular culture. After 2 Live Crew sampled "me so horny, me love you long time" for their 1989 hit "Me So Horny," the phrase became an expression of true skankiness. Divorced from the context of Kubrick's film, the phrase spoken in broken English with an Asian accent stands in for the nasty Asian girl.[17]

The Director and one of the women are left alone on stage singing "All alone . . . / surrounded by newspaper. . . . / All alone . . . / with a plastic helicopter" to the orchestral theme of *Les Miserables*, a musical written by the same lyricist and composer who wrote *Miss Saigon*. The woman exits, leaving The Director alone on stage fawning over his toy helicopter. As the lights dim and "The Love Duet" from *Madama Butterfly* comes up, two women enter the stage. The two would-be prostitutes who strutted off stage in the previous scene make their return as prostitutes. One, dressed as The Ghost of Madame Butterfly in a purple kimono and an ill-fitting geisha wig, carries a large plastic knife. (After losing the original wig, one of the company members purchased the new wig at a costume shop complete with flowers and chopsticks built right into the hair. When the new wig appeared at rehearsal one evening, the cast oohed and aahed at both the ingenuity of the wig's completeness and the fact that the stereotype could be purchased.)

These few signifiers of "Japanese-ness" elicit a good deal of laughter from the audience; and the second woman reenters. Wearing a white *ao dai* while holding a toy gun, she doubles as Kim from *Miss Saigon*. Both women enter the space by walking through the holes in the newspaper curtain. The Ghost of Madame Butterfly walks downstage right, while Ms. Saigon walks on a parallel path, positioning herself downstage left. Mocking Western representations of Japanese femininity, The Ghost of Madame Butterfly walks with her knees bent, turning one foot in and then rotating it out as she takes each forward step toward the audience. Ms. Saigon walks forward in a straight line, albeit slowly and deliberately, putting one foot in front of the other.

Puccini's 1910 opera, *Madama Butterfly,* and its modern musical adaptation, *Miss Saigon,* are the obvious inspirations for The Ghost of Madame Butterfly and Ms. Saigon. Performing the most dramatic moments in both the opera and the musical, the two women stand side by side, with pained expressions on their faces. Both women slowly raise their weapons of choice: The Ghost of Madame Butterfly lifts her oversized, plastic hara-kiri knife, and Ms. Saigon, her toy pistol. Their hands tremble as they draw their weapons toward their torsos. The rest of the cast, who have crawled back to the edges of the stage to watch the dramatic moment, are hysterical, yelling phrases like, "It's so moving. The music is so beautiful." They cling to one another and stare, as if enraptured by what is about to happen. As the music builds and the action unfolds, the watching performers slowly rise off the floor, their bodies reaching toward the two women, as if they are about to jump out of their seats in anticipation of the women's acts of suicide. The two women are on the verge of committing the fatal act as the music reaches a crescendo, when Ms. Saigon, with her gun at her temple, screams, "Cut the music, cut the music!"

The lights come up, the music stops abruptly, and the performers watching the two women look around in confusion. Ms. Saigon throws her arms down, slouches her upper body, and crosses her arms in frustration, demanding to know where the White Guy is.[18] The Director gets up from the back of the stage where he was watching and tries to appease Ms. Saigon, while a confused Ghost of Madame Butterfly tries to stay in character:

Ms. Saigon: Where is The White Guy?

Director: What white guy?

Ms. Saigon: We need a White Guy!

Director: A white guy? What for?

Ms. Saigon: You know, to save us! [*beat*] I am *not* going to kill myself without . . . a White Guy.

Butterfly: Pinkerton? Pinkerton?

Ms. Saigon: Shut-up! Casting director, I want a White Guy, and I want him NOW!

Director: Ms. Saigon, please calm down. We're trying to look . . .

Ms. Saigon: Try harder! [*she threatens him with a gun*]

At the brink of narrative closure, Ms. Saigon steps out of character to play the demanding prima donna.

What follows is a series of twists on the narrative conventions inherited from the opera *Madama Butterfly*, represented by The Ghost of Madame Butterfly, whose presence on stage is a live referent to the character that embodies the stereotype. Ms. Saigon plays at being Miss Saigon, insisting on the impossibility of playing the role of herself without a white referent.

Unlike the Broadway version of *Miss Saigon,* in which the Filipino cast seeks to be seen as Vietnamese, the Vietnamese American performer playing Ms. Saigon performs the effort of performing as Ms. Saigon performing Miss Saigon. She brandishes her toy gun, frowns, and pouts as she demands the conditions under which the stereotype within the narrative can make sense.

The Ghost of Madame Butterfly standing opposite Ms. Saigon tries desperately to continue the narrative. She fidgets nervously, pats her hair, and flinches while Ms. Saigon screams at the Casting Director. Ms. Saigon finds Madame Butterfly annoying in her commitment to the role. When the Casting Director tells Ms. Saigon that he is having a hard time finding a white guy to play the role of A White Guy, Ms. Saigon continues to fume. The Casting Director then looks out into the audience and asks, "Is there a white guy in the house? We need A White Guy," making fun of the practice by which any Asian body can play any other Asian body as a backdrop. A White Guy becomes an object and anyone will do at the moment, since the important thing to remember is that Ms. Saigon and Madame Butterfly simply need the presence of A White Guy to complete the narrative that accompanies the climatic moment of their suicides.

Suddenly, an Asian man dressed in a leopard-print tank top and matching shorts leaps onto and rolls across the stage, yodeling like Tarzan. He approaches The Ghost of Madame Butterfly and proclaims:

Tarzan: Me Tarzan, you Jane?

Ms. Saigon: What is this? He's not white!

Tarzan: I can dye my hair blond.

Ms. Saigon: Director! This man is an impostor!

Director: Impostor!?

Tarzan: But, Director, white people play Asians in the movies all the time!

Ms. Saigon: Just get him back to the jungle where he belongs.

Director: [*To Tarzan*] You heard the lady. I'm sorry, but you're just not what we're looking for.

Tarzan: [*whining*] But, Director . . .

Director: I'm sorry, but this isn't Hollywood. This is (*name of a particular performance venue*). Please, don't call us, we'll call you.

Tarzan's entrance is unexpected, and the logic for his presence is convoluted. Tarzan—whose story is the subject of innumerable novels, feature-length films, and television series—is a white man who was raised by chimpanzees in an African jungle. This animal-like man is both at one with and a master of jungle animals and terrain. Coded as questionably brown and unquestionably white, Tarzan is more civilized than black Africans, but more masculine than the white colonists bent on destroying Tarzan's jungle.[19]

Tarzan tumbles on stage and scratches himself. With his knees bent and legs wide apart, he lopes and sniffs at the women. The Vietnam War is always depicted as jungle warfare in a literal jungle inhabited by stealthy and chameleonlike Vietcong soldiers who are indistinguishable from each other, civilians, and the landscape itself. While the role of Tarzan requires that the performer overplay the stereotype adeptly, Ms. Saigon reminds the performer playing Tarzan that he is not white and therefore cannot possibly portray A White Guy. The Casting Director reminds the performers that this is low-budget theater and thus unable to ascribe to the same practices as Hollywood—in this case, cross-racial casting. Given this parodic twist on logical reasoning, The Casting Director asserts that he will not cast a Vietnamese American in the role of Tarzan, because Tarzan the Apeman is traditionally played by a white male actor.

Ms. Saigon's insistence on Tarzan's unsuitability also intersects with the role's hypermasculinity and the emasculation of Asian male bodies. After the performer playing Tarzan leaves the stage as a dejected would-be Tarzan, he returns as Rambo, ready to save Ms. Saigon and Madame Butterfly from who knows what. The *Rambo* trilogy, produced between 1982 and 1989, glorifies the exploits of John J. Rambo, a highly trained Vietnam War veteran, who finds himself unappreciated and persecuted by local authorities in the first film and the U.S. government in the second and third films. Rambo operates as a one-person army, engaged in guerilla warfare with the local sheriff's office in small-town Oregon (*First Blood*); Vietnamese communists (*Rambo: First Blood Part II*); and Russian communists (*Rambo III*). In each film,

Rambo must fight against a corrupt U.S. authority who threatens to under-mine Rambo's attempt to win the war against communism, a struggle that identifies him as a true patriot. Rambo's superhuman ability to endure tor-ture at the hands of Vietnamese communists and to single-handedly win the war against the Russians for Afghanistan marks him as a wrongly perse-cuted, Christ-like figure.

Unlike Tarzan, Rambo is not rejected, but the action continues as Ms. Saigon cries, "Don't take me, take my son!" to which The Ghost of Madame Butterfly responds, "Don't take her, take me," and the two women start to bicker about who is going to go off with Rambo. "Vietnamese Rambo" is funny because he is a narrative impossibility: the male Vietnamese body is visually indistinguishable from the Vietcong body, always already naturalized and "at one" with the jungle (Tarzan-like). The Vietnamese male body does not need to overcome it through sheer force or unimaginable bravery. The jungle, real and imagined, is both an untamed, natural landscape and a lawless political environment that operates as a natural habitat for the Vietcong, who is both the wild animal that will strike at any moment and the soul of political corruption. The scene ends with an indifferent Vietnamese Rambo dragging Ms. Saigon and Madame Butterfly off stage. He has a difficult time with the full weight of both women clutching his legs, and he complains, "I thought Oriental women were supposed to be petite." Vietnamese Rambo finally makes it off stage despite all the extra baggage.

"THE GOOD GUYS"

The quick-paced appearance of filmic stereotypes segues into a more somber portrait of the mass media. "The Good Guys" employs dark humor to dra-matize an essay by Andrew Lam titled "Love, Money, Prison, Sin, Revenge." Originally published in the *Los Angeles Times Magazine* on March 13, 1994, the essay seeks to understand a tragedy that took place at a Good Guys electronics store in Sacramento, California, in the early 1990s. While Lam's essay makes connections between the effects of the Vietnam War and Viet-namese American youth, Club O' Noodles borrows from the text of Lam's essay to reenact the events of April 4, 1991, as a meditation on representations of Vietnamese American youth in the media. Lam was unable to interview the four youths (all were between the ages of sixteen and twenty-one at the time)—Loi Khac Nguyen, Pham Khac Nguyen, Long Khac Nguyen, and

Cuong Tran—but in his attempt to understand them Lam interviewed their families and friends. To retell the story from within the crime scene, Club O' Noodles weaves excerpts from the interviews in Lam's essay to recreate the events of the shooting. The cast of characters in the "The Good Guys" includes the three brothers and their friend (who are mistaken as four brothers) and The Sheriff, all of whom are based on individuals central to the original headlines in 1991. To this cast, Club O' Noodles adds a new character, a Vietnamese American female reporter named Ugen Nugen, who grossly mispronounces her own name.

Four prerecorded gunshots startle the audience and the actors playing The Brothers storm onto the stage with their hostages. Two Brothers push The Hostages to the ground, while the other two threaten The Hostages as well as the audience with their weapons. The audience laughs when they see that the weapons are really toilet bowl cleaners, car clubs, plungers, feather dusters, and a variety of other household items. With The Hostages lying face down on the ground and The Brothers standing over them ready to beat or "shoot" them with their "weapons," it is not yet clear what the violence is referring to. Like other scenes, this one sets up the expectation that it is a reference to the Vietnam War, especially when the character Mai yells, "Shut the fuck up! Or I shoot you like fucking Vietcong." But unlike the previous piece, the spoof is not funny.

Everyone on stage freezes in place and a spotlight focuses on the woman who is playing Ugen Hugen. She adjusts her beige sports coat, chats with an imaginary cameraman, clears her throat, then peers into the audience to deliver her report. "On the afternoon of April 4, 1991—fifteen years, eleven months, and twenty-seven days after the end of the Vietnam War—four Vietnamese youths armed with semiautomatic weapons stormed into a Good Guys electronics store and held forty-one people hostage. Speaking in heavily accented and broken English, they issued what the sheriff has described as a 'series of bizarre demands.' "[20]

Playing upon the media's inability to distinguish between different Asian groups, The Reporter misreports what is happening at the crime site. By performing the constructedness of the news media, she plays up the distance between herself and the subject that she is reporting. The actors portraying The Four Brothers also exaggerate the "bizarre" circumstances that characterized the news reports.

Hiep: Du ma! We want revenge!

Hung: Yeah we want a *real* helicopter to fly to Thailand.

Hiep: We want to kill all fucking communists who ruin our family!
I want revenge for my father!

Journey: We want four million dollars!

Hung: Four bulletproof vests!

Mai: And lots of 1000-year-old ginseng root!

Hiep: Do it now! Or we will start killing the white people one by
one! [*Everyone freezes.*][21]

"The Good Guys" re-presents how the media reported the crime and not
what actually happened. The work makes fun of the disjuncture between
The Reporter and the suspects, even though both are sharing the same space
on stage. The Reporter is portrayed as a Connie Chung–like figure, whose
behavior also calls into question the idea that an Asian American reporter is
going to somehow give more authentic information about a crime involving
Asian American suspects. She continues to mispronounce The Brothers'
names and reports that they all speak heavily accented and broken English.
Ironically, the four performers playing The Brothers deliver their lines in
both English and Vietnamese. Some of them imitate Vietnamese accents
when they speak English, while others do not.

The culmination of the scene is a powerful monologue delivered by the
male actor playing Hiep. By now, one of the hostages has tried to leave the
stage, and Hiep has "shot" him in the back with his feather duster. More
gunshots ring out, and all of The Brothers fall to the ground except for Hiep.
A disembodied voice addresses Hiep, who falls to his knees when a bright
spotlight shines directly into his eyes. Unable to differentiate between Hiep's
first and last names, The Sheriff asks, "Mr. Hiep, are you or are you not a
gangster?" Hiep crumbles to the ground, looks at the audience, and replies:

I want America to notice me. At night, I see other Vietnamese kids
wander the streets like ghosts. Some run away from home. Some
have no homes to run from. Some just roam from one city to another
. . . looking for something . . . not knowing what. . . . People think

that I'm just a stupid pig . . . that I'm just a nobody. I came to this country as a Vietnamese refugee, the son of a South Vietnamese army officer. My brothers and I, through our father . . . are veterans of a civil war we never fought. We cry for vengeance. Why? Because to grow up in America is to want fame and glory. America does not want losers! Here, history is already against us. Vietnam goes on without us. America goes on without acknowledging us. I don't want to be beside the point, a footnote in some history book. . . .[22]

Hiep's eloquent speech is interrupted by The Sheriff, who asks, "Are you or aren't you a gangster?" Repeated by the disembodied voice, the question becomes a meaningless soundscape disengaged from what Hiep is saying, from Hiep himself. It is as if The Sheriff and his questions are a tape recording, unable to respond any differently when faced with the sight of a young Vietnamese male body.

The Reporter returns to the stage, gestures to an invisible cameraperson, and performs being on camera. She reports, "A swat team raided the store eight and a half hours later. Three of the young gunmen were killed immediately, but not before one of them sprayed the hostages with bullets—killing three and wounding eight. Hiep Ne Gu Gen, the oldest, was seriously wounded. His trial of forty-nine felony counts and three counts of murder is set for July 11. This is Ugen Hugen, reporting from Little Saigon, for k-pho Channel 99. Now a word from our sponsor."[23] She then takes a commercial break and everyone involved in the scene starts to sing "Be all that you can be . . . in the Army"—an ironic reference to the very military structure that was used to create the situation that Hiep described in his monologue. The irony of living in the country that was trying to kill you is not lost.

Following Rambo, The Brothers take on the identity of the disillusioned Vietnam War vet fighting against persecution by the police. But Ms. Saigon has already pointed out that The Brothers inhabit problematic Asian bodies. Unlike the filmic Rambo, whose one-man military exploits represent the ultimate expression of patriotism, The Brothers' requests are framed as random and ridiculous. Their desire for military revenge falls outside of the imagination of U.S. military-as-cultural interests, even though the Vietnam War–based narrative offers the public a guaranteed premise for action-packed Hollywood filmic entertainment.

FINALE

In *Laughter's* final scene, the audience is presented with a ritual setting. The woman playing the role of Ms. Saigon opens the final act singing Trịnh Công Sơn's anti-war folk song, "Gia tài của mẹ" (A Mother's Heritage) in Vietnamese, while a male performer stands on the opposite side of the stage reciting an English translation of the lyrics.[24] Everyone else walks hunched across the stage. In canon, they slowly raise their upper bodies until standing in an upright position, a phrase reminiscent of the opening scene. The rest of the cast joins in the singing, while each performer gathers newspaper to build a large mound in the middle of the stage. One by one, the cast members disappear offstage and re-enter carrying the straw hats used in "From War to Hollywood." This time the hats don't elicit giggles, as the cast lines up alongside the mound. The soloist and her translator stand at the head of the mound and bow facing the grave. The stage set has turned into a gravesite; one of the performers recalls the fairy tale told at the very beginning of the performance:

> Legend has it that the children of the Dragon Prince and the Fairy Princess who had run away, once lost and confused, now have found homes in places like Westminster, California, Houston, Texas, and even in Little Rock, Arkansas. They create a new family. They learn to sing a new song, and dance a new dance. Searching for a new language, they begin to tell stories, the stories of the children of war.

Taking turns, each performer states his or her full name and birth date, then grabs a handful of shredded paper from his or her hat and throws it on the mound. They each recite one final line and exit the stage.

In this scene, the performers claim the ability to invent a new identity. Incense, along with the couple bowing in prayer at one end of the gravelike mound, evokes religious images of ancestor worship. This scene reiterates the visual image of newspaper piles from the beginning of the performance, but this time the pile is one gigantic mound instead of ten separate ones. It is a surprise that the performance ends with a ritual reminiscent of traditional Vietnamese funerals, since most of the performance departs from, or is a comment on, what "Vietnamese" is. This is also a moment when the performers draw attention to their own identities outside of the context of the performance. This shift from portraying a character to that of naming one-self as an individual becomes dramatic and significant. The audience hears the performers' birth dates—1969, 1979, 1972, 1975—to remind them of an era simply referred to as "Vietnam" in the United States. Vietnamese Americans are no longer a footnote in U.S. history books, because, all of a sudden, they are on stage as individualized bodies announcing their presence attached to the legacy of the war in Vietnam.

Form and Popular Culture

One of the most striking features of Club O' Noodles's work is its extensive citation of popular culture; however, it is important to point out that the artists themselves do not think of their work as popular culture. Club O' Noodles's references to popular culture are reminiscent of Dan Kwong's parody of New Age gurus in *Monkhood in Three Easy Lessons* and Denise Uyehara's satirical take on stand-up comedy and Hello Kitty products in *Hello (Sex) Kitty*. In these artists' works, popular culture operates as a foil that the protagonist must work against in order to recuperate Asian American subjectivity and agency.

By making pop cultural references within a nonlinear narrative, Club O' Noodles is able to situate its work within recognizable historical moments, such that a reference to *Gilligan's Island* evokes the 1970s, an all-American childhood, and childhood memories of escape from war. The scene itself has nothing to do with *Gilligan's Island* in terms of specific characters or plots, other than the general reference to shipwreck and open seas—and yet, because *Laughter* includes both *Gilligan's Island* and "Boat Dance," the company creates layers of meaning. This is a different approach to evoking time and space than that of an artist like Ping Chong, who situates his own work squarely in the realm of high-art avant-gardism. Although Chong complicates time, space, and bodies by using cross-racial casting, his work relies on the presentation of a series of identifiable historical moments performed through historical characters in roughly chronological order.[25] For example, in *Deshima*, each discrete scene in the performance alludes to specific moments in Japanese history. Although the scenes may skip centuries from one moment to another, a narrator announces to the audience that "time passes" between the scenes. Chong references what would be ambiguous moments in

Japanese history (ambiguous for U.S. audiences) with narrative clarity, while Club O' Noodles uses the familiar language of popular culture to stage overlapping spaces and time.

Club O' Noodles choreographs identities on stage by using the body's ability to say one thing while doing another, within a theatrical frame that calls attention to the competing discourses of artifice and authenticity. The theatrical frame allows Club O' Noodles's performers to mix fictional characters with those based on themselves. Club O' Noodles is also working from the space of activist performance and postmodern dance—practices invested in notions of authenticity, self-authorship, and community. These themes appear in *Laughter* as the performers' bodies evoke multiple locations both temporal and geographic within the same moment, while the stories presented are rooted in autobiographical memories and channeled through popular culture.

Leaving the Theater

After attending Club O' Noodles's performance at Highways Performance Space, I left the theater with a book of notes scribbled in the dark. My notes record the pleasure of seeing a performance unfold for the first time and the rush of adrenaline when so many things are happening on stage simultaneously that it is difficult to write them all down. These notes include the details and reactions that I no longer saw or felt during subsequent viewings, not because the material itself had changed but because, in the first performance, I had felt the surprise and delight that comes with not knowing what will happen next. Dorinne Kondo writes about the pleasure offered by performance; however, I found in making performance the object of study, pleasure disappeared as I returned to the theater with the researcher's critical eye. The prospect of performance as research changed my approach to viewing. Gone was the faith in letting a performance wash over my senses, as I began to look for and anticipate structures and narratives. I could be disappointed but not surprised if that which I was looking for was not there; approving but not moved if it was. Once performance itself became the representative object to be interpreted, not experienced, I found myself narrating my analysis in the dark before the performance was over.

After the first night I saw *Laughter,* I left Highways with a business card, a rehearsal date, and a set of directions—not knowing I would be attending workshops, traveling, and performing with Club O' Noodles for the next three years. Chapter 3, "Rehearsing the Collective: A Performative Autoethnography," recounts a bodily engagement with *Laughter* outside the context of the staged performance. Looking at Club O' Noodles's rehearsal process extends the boundaries of *Laughter* to consider the significance of what does or does not make it into staged productions. The following chapter analyzes how Club O' Noodles crafts its own identity as a Vietnamese American performance collective that is both in concert with and in contradiction to the representations offered by their staged productions.

3

REHEARSING THE COLLECTIVE
A Performative Autoethnography

After attending Club O' Noodles's performance of *Laughter,* I approached Hung Nguyen, the artistic director of the company, about coming to a rehearsal and interviewing the members of the group about the show. "Sure, come and play," was Nguyen's reply. Armed with a rented video camera and a newly purchased notepad for the occasion, I trekked across the Southern California freeway system to begin my dissertation research, but Nguyen never said, "Sure, come and begin your dissertation research." He had said, "Sure, come and play." Play, or more precisely, participate, was what I was asked and expected to do.

For this reason, I call this work a performative autoethnography to account for the research methodology used to gather research data on Club O' Noodles. Over the course of a three-year period, my "play" with the collective grew increasingly participatory, to such an extent that I found a need to grapple with the frameworks of anthropological discourse and critiques of anthropology. I am suspicious of ethnographic methods and writing, even though the actual techniques I employed to collect information (participation/observation, informal interviews, video documentation, and taking field notes) are trademarks of anthropological work. The suspicion lies in the realization that an ethnography about Club O' Noodles's rehearsal process is not a tell-all about backstage life, but selected fragments of a working process.

At the 2001 Asian American Studies Conference in Toronto, Dan Bacalzo delivered a paper about the New York–based performance ensemble Peeling the Banana. In his talk, Bacalzo described the ways in which the artists performed alternative representations of Asian American subjectivity that challenged normative understandings of gender and sexuality. When he was asked how one "ignores one's presence" within a performance as either a performer or a director, the discussion turned toward the politics of writing ethnographically and "airing dirty laundry." The issue of airing dirty laundry illustrates the need for further contextualization in terms of representational betrayal within the seemingly conflicting disciplines of anthropology and Asian American studies.[1] Namely, anthropology's colonial past is that of a subjugating practice of representing non-Western and non-white peoples as other, versus the self-representational rhetoric opposing processes of othering that informs Asian American studies. A performative autoethnographer attempts to foreground her own subjective position as scholar, performer, and Chinese American woman doing research on Club O' Noodles. It reveals a research methodology (ethnography), subject position (auto), and the inherent problems in claiming a subject position (authority, subject as object, researcher/researched) within ethnographic writing. It is a "performative" autoethnography because it addresses the following:

1. Performance as ethnography, whereby the process of generating material for CON's performances is a form of ethnographic research and its staged productions are performed ethnographic representations.
2. My participation in the rehearsal and performance processes as well as how the research I performed (writing notes, taping rehearsals, interviewing) in the field is translated into a written account.
3. The question of power within ethnographic writing and the denaturalization of the native in native anthropology.

In raising the question of representational power on the part of the ethnographer, this narrative is still motivated by a desire to understand what it means for a self-identified Vietnamese American performance ensemble to "rehearse" an identity if that ensemble's staged production is indeed a choreography of identity.

Is it a ludicrous question to consider whether one rehearses an identity as if one were practicing scales or perfecting a double pirouette? I wanted to understand what technique is involved in creating a show about Vietnamese America, in order to think concretely about the making of Asian American performance studies. Working from the space of Asian American studies offered me numerous models for thinking reflexively about the issue of representation in ethnographic writing; therefore, this performative auto-ethnography draws on Johannes Fabian's and Dorinne Kondo's conceptualizations of performative ethnography.

Performative Ethnography: Fabian and Kondo

In his study of the popular theater troupe Groupe Mufwankolo in Shaba, Zaïre, Fabian characterizes the watching of staged performance as "communicative exchanges" that involve both performer and ethnographer (1990, 11–12). Thus, staged productions are not only "texts" to be read by the viewer, but an interactive exchange between what happens on stage and on the body of the viewer (and in this case, the viewer is the ethnographer). He frames theatrical performance as a form of ethnographic representation and his own writing about performed ethnographies as performative rather than informative ethnography. Staged performances, like ethnographic writing, are events through which information is transferred between performer and ethnographer and are not information in and of itself.[2] The shift to conceptualizing information as movement disrupts the notion that the performance of a theatrical production is a discrete object.

In resisting the temptation to see staged performances as the "final product" and thus "finite meaning," Fabian looks to the rehearsal process as a generative space for producing meaning. It may seem obvious to consider rehearsal space as a necessary component of studying performance, but, within the context of Western theatrical dance, rehearsal is distinctly separate from the staged performances. Open rehearsals and dress rehearsals often blur this distinction, but these events are not the complete performance itself in terms of temporal and spatial locations. It is understood that the staged performance is fair game for a final evaluation as a "performed object," while rehearsal is not. Since the 1960s, postmodern choreographers in the United States have championed the ethos of "process-over-product" as a way of challenging the notion of what is the dance. Cynthia Novack's treatment of contact improvisation echoes this sentiment. Novack characterizes contact improvisation as a form emerging from a white avant-garde art scene that most closely approximates a form of "communal dance" (1990).

A dancer's view of contact improvisation as a lifestyle is akin to the way researchers generally characterize dance in African societies as lacking separation from everyday life. That dancing in the United States is considered an activity separate from everyday life is a given, and narratives of dance as ritual, religion, and so on have provided a narrative of cultural utopia for dancers and dance scholars. In this utopia, one dances all day, creating a population fully integrated in mind, body, and spirit. My point here is not to argue whether or not this is true, but to situate where this ethnography is not going in terms of following Fabian's move into the rehearsal space. Club O' Noodles's work is clearly produced for the proscenium stage, but its self-identified contribution as an organization lies in the rehearsal process. The challenge here resides in representing the proximity of the rehearsal process to the stage production without succumbing to a discourse that naturalizes ethnography as the obvious means for studying non-white cultural productions and process-over-product as a way of framing community-based performance.

To resist the reification of the final product, Fabian looks to rehearsal as an equally important source of communicative exchange, while maintaining a hard distinction between staged performance and rehearsal. He is careful to recognize the significance of each category in terms of how it functions differently within the larger public sphere. Fabian accomplishes this differentiation in order to de-hierarchize the relationship between the observer (the ethnographer) and the observed (the studied subject) within ethnographic writing as one specific sphere. Since his studied subjects (the performers) already "have a voice" in that they are publicly producing theatrical productions aired on national television in Zaïre, Fabian claims that he can only represent his own process of instigating a collective attempt (between himself and Groupe Mufwankolo) to answer his question via a theatrical production on the subject of the phrase *le pouvoir se mange entier* (power is eaten whole).

On the afternoon of that day in 1986 I had brought it up when I met with a group of popular actors whom I had known since the seventies. I did this with no particular purpose in mind and I was overwhelmed by their eagerness to explain "le pouvoir se mange entier" to me and to themselves. Spontaneously they decided that it would be just the right topic for their next play. On the spot they began planning—first suggestions for a plot were made, problems of translating the French term *pouvoir* were debated, several actors cited sayings and customs from their home country—in short, I had triggered an ethnographic brainstorm. (3)

In mapping out a matrix of meaning, Fabian's subjects, the actors themselves, are not reduced to culturally essentialized bodies of knowledge, whereby knowledge is a fixed entity that can be possessed; knowledge is, instead, a negotiation between people. Within this understanding of cultural knowledge, Fabian's "native informants" are not approached as repositories of truths that can be observed and recorded, but Fabian attends to the actors' process of translating cultural knowledge from one form to another. In this case—during the entire period from Fabian's question to the actual theatrical production—Fabian never provides the reader an answer to his question; or, at most, he answers with the narrative of a process.

Fabian observes that Groupe Mufwankolo's final performance-as-product did not reflect the range of possible answers generated during the rehearsal process. To account for the relationship between performance and rehearsal, he maintains that rehearsal is part of the performance but is not a substitute for performance; while performance cannot truly represent the rehearsal process, yet it is the final performance that is televised as "the representation." Both are dependent upon one another.

An image that keeps coming up as I think about the texts and performances around the theme "le pouvoir se mange entier" to which this study is devoted is that of an iceberg. Performance is the visible tip; rehearsal/repetition the submerged body. Such a spatial or corporeal image may at first seem an inappropriate evocation of process yet it helps to clarify an important insight. As the tip of the iceberg does not represent its submerged part, cultural performances do not symbolize the work of repetition and rehearsal. They are *carried* by that work; there is an unbroken, material connection which is metonymic, not metaphoric. As far as I can see, process can—productively—only be conceived of metonymically. (12)

A staged performance is not a symbol of culture but, rather, an enactment of knowledge that is part of a social dialogue that continues in a time and space designated as "not the performance itself." Using a spatial/corporeal meta-phor in order to liken ethnography to what he calls a "repetition of perfor-mances," Fabian claims that culture at any given time can be witnessed in the form of "a tip of the iceberg," which is not a symbol of the entire submerged body. Staged performance is a "part, a moment of a process" of the rehearsal-as-repetition, but not the rehearsal itself (12).

Fabian sees Groupe Mufwankolo's performances as a kind of "per-formed ethnography" like that of his own ethnographic writing. The rehear-sal process is the shared encounter between the ethnographer and the actors as they attempt to translate the meaning of *le pouvoir se mange entier* from one form to another. This performative ethnography assumes coevalness be-tween himself and the subject of study. He writes:

> Informative ethnography—collecting data and information about another culture—corresponds to a political situation of more or less direct control, one in which the ethnographer as the emissary of the dominant power (wittingly or not) has the upper hand; where he or she can ask the questions, determine what counts as information, control the situations in which it is to be gathered, and so forth. Performative ethnography—the kind where the ethnographer does not call the tune but plays along—would be the approach that fits situations where our societies no longer exercise direct control. (19)

Fabian's epistemological point of departure assumes a coevalness between himself and Groupe Mufwankolo, or at least a diminishing of his authorial presence in his writing. The significance of his theoretical move is relative to a reader's preconceived notions of his authority. Although Fabian claims to "do ethnography with, not of Groupe Mufwankolo" (43), the reader has no sense of Fabian as a character within his ethnography. He is inquisitive, insightful, and sophisticated, without any quirks or faults—but his infor-mants provide the action of the story. His theoretical move from informative to performative ethnography does not quite translate into a reflection on himself as a subject. For him to share authority does not ruin his project, which suggests that the body of the researcher is, in fact, more important than Fabian's rhetorical claim that the ethnographer is a body in dialogue with the performers.

In contrast to Fabian's approach to a performative ethnography, Dorinne Kondo takes up the question of subject position and the body of the ethnographer from an altogether different place. Like Fabian, Kondo frames theatrical performance as ethnographic practice. Unlike Fabian, she takes on a subject position not just as an ethnographer in relationship to her subject, but also as an ethnographer with a racial, gender, and national identity that affects her relationship to her subjects. Kondo claims proximity to her subjects not so much for the purpose of revealing dialogic exchanges between researcher and researched, but to produce her own identity as an anthropologist, an Asian American woman, and a scholar/activist. In 1997's *About Face*, she writes:

> Certainly, "going home"—not only to *study* one's own community, with all the asymmetries of power that term implies, but also to help *create* it—gives one a wholly different relationship to the usual anthropological project of distanced observation and studying down. The distant ethnographer/observer can become a participant fully engaged in a common struggle of great political urgency, in which we can contribute as much as we receive. (205; emphasis in original)

While Fabian negotiates distance between researcher and researched, Kondo —in order to circumvent the question of power relationships—also claims a racial, ethnic, and political affinity with the Japanese designers and Asian American playwrights she writes about.

Kondo's proximity to her subject focuses on "Asian American" as a shared political identity mediated through Orientalism. Japanese fashion designers working in a predominantly European and American design community are subject to the same stereotypes as Asian American students protesting a production of *The Mikado* on a college campus. For Kondo, Japanese national identity and Asian American political identity are both constructed in relationship to Western representations of Asian bodies as a racial category. Kondo claims a "native" subject position as a coalitional move and identifies with Japanese American and Chinese American playwrights under the rubric of a universalized Asian American identity.

Kondo's ethnographic approach allows her readers a glimpse of who attends Asian American performances and what kinds of venues produce them. She presents multiple approaches to writing about what can be considered Asian American performance; these include her reaction to Perry Mi-yake's play *Doughball*, an interview with playwright David Henry Hwang, and an ethnographic account of a public protest against *Miss Saigon*. Kondo's presence in the text extends beyond reporting observations and includes accounts of how she sees herself as a key player in influencing theater. Thus, she sets forth a series of disruptions regarding the traditional role of the anthropologist and ethnographic writing.

Kondo does not necessarily write about her bodily presence. Her body is inferred. The reader gets an idea of how Kondo attempts to broker change by using her position and skills in a way that might generate attention for her subject outside of academic writing for other intellectuals. She gives her readers (intellectuals, no doubt) concrete examples of how one might evince social change by calling attention to the academic's access to power. She never refers to the specific power of the researcher over the subject. She deals with multiple topics, on which she is constantly shifting her perspective between insider and outsider, representer and represented. She also charges the "na-tive anthropologists" with a new challenge—not just simply to "get it right," but to continuously create that which is new. There is not necessarily an "old" that functions as an antagonist to the "new," but I use "new" to demarcate the researcher's sense of engaging in invention rather than "reporting what has happened." I am alluding to the possibility of writing that identifies with mobilization—actual movement through space, moving from one idea to another, and social change.

Kondo creates a sense of mobilization by connecting seemingly different topics in a rhizomatic manner (Deleuze and Guattari, 1980). Her narrative begins with the specificity of her attendance at a haute couture fashion show, followed by a close analysis of fashion magazines read at an unspecified time and place. What appears to be the most apolitical and frivolous stage, the fashion show, proves to be a high-powered arena where race and nation are clearly demarcated through costuming. She then takes our attention to the marginalized stage of Asian American theater as a site of intervention. For example, she demonstrates the impossibility of thinking about Asian Ameri-can theater without David Henry Hwang's *M. Butterfly* coming to mind. And to think about *M. Butterfly,* one must consider *Miss Saigon* and *Madama Butterfly*. And to do that, we are brought back to the larger issue of Japan, how Japanese-ness is circulating globally, and the contradiction between Western discourses of Japan and Japan as a colonizing force in Southeast Asia. There is an unfinished quality about the scope of the topics she addresses, which indirectly names the impossible task of accounting for all the ways in which Orientalism comes into play.

Kondo's relationship to each subject changes. Sometimes she is the outsider (the fashion show), the insider (audience member at Asian American play, protester at the opening of *Miss Saigon*), the authority (author of a book, author of a protest letter to the *Los Angeles Times*), or the represented (protester of *Miss Saigon*, audience member of Perry Miyake's production of *Doughball*). Her power relationship to her subject of study is constantly shifting. Her choice of the multibillion-dollar fashion industry complicates the notion that a researcher goes into the field and leaves with the upper hand in terms of the ability to represent a subject. Obviously, the fashion industry shapes what the world should want to think about, look like, live like, and be like. This is also true of the theater industry, as she writes in her protest of *Miss Saigon*. Despite the controversy regarding both the casting and the content of the musical, it continues to be performed to sold-out audiences all over the world and to exist unscathed in terms of its popular and economic success. Kondo's relationship to the Asian American playwrights and play texts also muddles easy classification of her subject position. She writes about the Tony award–winning *M. Butterfly*, but she is also instrumental in drawing attention to a play like Perry Miyake's *Doughball*. In describing her motivations for writing about *Doughball*, Kondo states:

> Small wonder I experience this play with almost physical force, in my whole being. Small wonder I spent the subsequent week in a fog, musing about the place of Stanford and of France as utopian landscapes for Sansei girls. And small wonder that mainstream critics were unable to understand the play fully. Instead of exoticism, they were exposed to the less spectacular, but infinitely more resonant, small truths of everyday life: the truths of home. As I felt with *M. Butterfly*, I was consumed by urgency to write about this play, to document its resonance, for never in my life have I seen anything so "true" to "my experience." (1997, 195)

By choosing to "document its resonance," she creates a different set of criteria on which to base her critique. The everyday is a different everyday, though it is the everyday just the same. Kondo herself becomes the subject of the play within her own writing about a play in which she recognizes herself for the first time.

My use of performative autoethnography merges Fabian's interest in the move from the informative to the performative and Kondo's insertion of herself as a subject of ethnography. In what might be viewed as a theoretical step backward, moving away from a metaphorical use of the term "performance" as a practice of everyday life, I am interested in taking a close look at how the everyday performances of identity that occur in rehearsals and workshops make their way into theatricalized representations of identity. Regardless of what happens during rehearsal, it is always in the service of a pending performance date. Performers do invent in the moment on stage, but also prepare elsewhere. Charged with the role of unfixing identities, repairing misrepresentations, educating, exposing ambiguities, and defining community on stage, ethnically identified performance events must work with what performance theorist José Muñoz (2000) refers to as "disidentification." Defined as "neither an identification nor a counter-identification—it is a working on, with, and against a form at a simultaneous moment."[3] In reference to Latino/a theater in the United States, Muñoz uses the concept of disidentification, rather than identification, as a way for queer Latinos/as in the United States to negotiate their relationships to clichés and stereotypes without succumbing to a practice of fixing one's identity through naming (70).

I would argue that theatrical performances mark, to a certain degree, one end point of the rehearsal, but this does not mean that performances do not provoke differing interpretations or that performances fix identity. The desire to read live theatrical performances by artists of color as ongoing explorations of identity is understandable, since live performance allows for the simultaneous staging of multiple identities.[4] Following Muñoz, the process of disidentifying and the act of representing a disidentification are two different activities. To give the performance-as-object all the credit for being a manifestation of disidentification (through textual analysis), rather than grappling with the process, erases the agency of the very body that is supposedly doing the disidentifying.

In the rest of this chapter, I present a number of ethnographic anecdotes that point toward specific moments during Club O' Noodles's rehearsals when the members make disidentifications with pan–Asian American and Vietnamese American identity politics and with the larger pan–Asian American performance and activist communities, then I describe how these are transformed into material for actual theatrical productions. Performative autoethnography is also a strategy I developed to account for considering aesthetic concerns within the process of writing about disidentification. In the previous chapter, I advocate for the idea that it is imperative to move beyond sociological interpretations of Asian American performance.[5] This is not a call for aesthetic neutrality, nor do I claim that Asian American bodies on stage can be separated from racialized discourses that "see" Asian-ness as a visible marker of racial-as-cultural identity.

Parody, satire, and campy performances of Orientalist stereotypes are common representative strategies used by contemporary Asian American performance artists to comment on the absurdities and harmfulness of racial stereotypes.[6] David Henry Hwang's *M. Butterfly* has been the topic of numerous articles by Asian American scholars arguing for or against the play's ability to disrupt the Madame Butterfly stereotype.[7]

Rather than focusing only on the success or failure of a particular representation, my performative autoethnography attends to the ways in which Club O' Noodles's theatrical performances represent agreements and compromises worked out between the performers prior to a stage production. For the performers, the performance is, in practice, an agreed-upon representation (at least for the moment) of the process of disidentification. This representation is born out of arguments and debates over the effectiveness of representational strategies (realism, parody, satire, abstraction, metaphor, and postmodern choreographic strategies) and aesthetic choices (what kinds of movement vocabulary, music, and text are used and how they are put together)—not all of which make it onto the stage. The following anecdote is an example of how disidentifications are negotiated through choreography, and how performers attempt to predict readings of their representations. This is not meant to establish authorial intent as the voice of authority, but to examine the struggle of creating self-representations within a representational field that always already signifies the material body.

In the winter of 1997, Club O' Noodles was scheduled to perform *Laughter from the Children of War* at a number of venues in California, including a couple of museums. Bernard, a stunt choreographer, was invited to redirect a fight scene in *Laughter*, because there had been several casting changes due to a turnover in the ensemble's membership since *Laughter* was first produced. This caused a certain degree of messiness in one fight scene, because the remaining original cast members could only remember parts of the choreography.

After introducing the group to a series of warm-ups, followed by a brief lesson in basic skills, Bernard began to set the choreography by giving specific directions to the performers. The following is an approximation of the stage directions that Bernard gave to the group before he was interrupted by Hung, the artistic director:

1. Uyen jumps on top of Ham, and Phuong punches Journey.
2. Thuc Nhi approaches Journey from behind, taps him on the shoulder and Journey turns around and dances with Thuc Nhi.
3. Phuong pushes Journey out of her way and fights with Thuc Nhi.

While Phuong and Thuc Nhi were in the middle of marking their fistfight, Hung stopped the action and objected to Bernard's casting. Hung claimed that it was not "politically correct for the two women to fight over a man." Afraid that audiences would interpret the fight—which, in the context of the performance, is supposed to be symbolic of war and alienation—as two jealous women fighting over a boyfriend, Hung tried to come up with a better visual solution, but the number and gender of the bodies available for casting complicated the situation.

Ideally, the fight scene immediately follows the hip-hop dance sequence performed in unison, leading into a reprise of a Vietnamese lullaby requiring the entire cast to be on stage. At this particular rehearsal, only five cast members were available to perform in the scene and Hung wanted to have at least one trio in the choreography to avoid the repetitiveness of too many duets. With two men and three women, the trio could only be cast as two men and one woman, or two women and one man. In order to accommodate a male/female duet that was supposed to happen simultaneously behind the trio, Hung did not considered the option of casting three women in a trio.

The difficulty with choreographing the trio occurred once Hung analyzed the choreography within a gendered narrative. He did not want two men fighting with one woman, thinking it would be interpreted as a gang rape, and he did not want too many combinations of two women fighting each other. Hung and Bernard finally settled, through compromise, that Phuong, Thuc Nhi, and Journey would form a trio. Phuong and Thuc Nhi throw a few punches at each other until Thuc Nhi finally collapses. Phuong then fights with Journey, whom she ends up throwing to the ground.

It is both an aesthetic and a political compromise based on the number of bodies present on stage and the implied narrative generated by visibly gendered bodies. To avoid a homogeneous use of space, the director uses both duets and trios, while the gendered narrative is made a bit more ambiguous with Phuong, who remains the last person standing. The rest have been thrown or have fallen to the ground. Not entirely convinced that the trio works, Hung changes the choreography in later productions when more cast members are available to perform. This particular combination of bodies within the choreography suited one particular performance and offered one particular representation open to the interpretation that Hung feared (two jealous women fighting over a two-timing boyfriend). The process is a struggle between a belief in allowing all the performers, regardless of gender or body size, the same movement vocabulary, and the gendered implications of that movement vocabulary in an actual performance. A close examination of the rehearsal process demonstrates how the members work through a multitude of choreographic choices in order to arrive at the least problematic representation.

This working out of gender for a theatrical performance happened in the rehearsal space, and the discussion of how gender is perceived began as a choreographic problem. The topic of gender was not foregrounded in this particular section of the performance, but presented itself during the rehearsal process because of the material presence of the bodies at a given time. Although the representation may "fail" in terms of producing an irrefutably transgressive representation of gender, the performers did explore the choreographic limits of the representational moment. My description is offered not as an excuse for making "bad" artistic choices, but to further Fabian's and Kondo's conceptualizations of performative ethnography and to consider an analysis of techniques used to create performances, to provide windows into the political and artistic compromises that must sometimes be made, and to reveal the schisms that sometimes must occur between artistic motives and the performance.

Checking In/Checking Out

Choreographically, Club O' Noodles draws on postmodern dance vocabularies and choreographic strategies to provide a space for aesthetic experimentation and to maintain an atmosphere of inclusiveness. The democratic principles proposed by postmodern choreographers and the focus on process-over-product in Club O' Noodles's rehearsals and workshops create a sense of community among its membership. In the late '90s, their rehearsal process was unique because it did not resemble the traditional notion of rehearsing a work. Instead of dedicating each meeting to work on material directly related to an upcoming performance or a work-in-progress, most often the company would devote a good portion of the rehearsal process to establishing cohesive relationships between the members through movement improvisations and discussions of personal feelings about issues related to individual as well as group identity.

The members of the group bracketed their membership by unsaid but understood racial and ethnic identities (which I will discuss later), so the rehearsal/workshop functioned as a space to work out issues of becoming an artist and, furthermore, asserting one's identity as an artist—in a modernist sense. Club O' Noodles's meetings were viewed as a place where the doing of artistic work was valued and supported by a community—the organization itself. Since many of the members viewed themselves as emerging artists, they viewed recognition and support from other artists differently from recognition by an audience. Supportive audiences served an important function as potential sources of future members. KCAL 9 News interviewed members of Club O' Noodles during the run of *Laughter from the Children of War* at the South Coast Repertory in Orange County, California. During the interview, Mai, who was a relatively new member at the time, told reporters that he had always wanted to be a professional actor but had felt self-conscious about his Vietnamese accent until he joined Club O' Noodles and found acceptance. What Mai alluded to indirectly is the social stigma associated with Asian accents that are represented by Hollywood and network television. That Mai's critique of casting practices found its way into the news broadcast is ironic given Club O' Noodles's critique of the media in *Laughter.*

Mai, who received a B.F.A. in theater studies from a large public university in Southern California, later claimed that he was never sure if the reason he was not cast in departmental productions had to do with his Vietnamese accent or if he was really just a bad actor. From the standpoint of the Asian American cultural critic, the answer to his question would appear obvious: directors did not cast him because had an Asian rather than a European accent.

Mai's question might sound naïve given the literature in Asian American studies on Hollywood casting practices, but I encountered the same question on a number of other occasions. In the summer of 1997, I participated in a two-week performance workshop taught by Tim Miller and Ping Chong, titled "Performance and the Other." Sometime during the second week of the workshop, Tim Miller asked each participant to discuss why she or he was attending the workshop. I talked about my work with Club O' Noodles and my interest in how the members viewed the organization as a place of refuge for Vietnamese American actors, dancers, singers, and writers who felt otherwise excluded from mainstream (white) art circles. A Korean woman came up to me during our break and said that she found my discussion of CON intriguing. She had earned her M.F.A. in theater studies from a (different) large public university in Southern California, and had often wondered why she was never cast in departmental productions. She thought maybe it was because she spoke with a Korean accent, but she was never certain and would spend time wondering if she was imagining things.

After relating my story to her, she felt somewhat vindicated, in the sense that she was finally able to name her experience and knew she had not imagined what had happened to her. This was especially important given the rhetoric of equal opportunity and meritocracy that U.S. educational institutions espouse. The woman had blamed herself for what she perceived as her personal failure because she did not know that what she experienced was also happening to other actors who sounded "too foreign." After graduation, the woman returned to Korea and became an important member of the theater scene in Seoul, where she was in charge of organizing a number of international theater festivals.

Club O' Noodles established itself as an artistically supportive space through a series of rituals, called "checking in" and "checking out," to mark the beginning and end of each meeting. Ideally, checking in occurred at the very beginning of a rehearsal to refocus everyone's attention on the present; checking out occurred at the end, to bring a meeting to a close and prepare everyone to meet again. Either the director or another designated person called for a check-in once s/he thought everyone who was going to show up for rehearsal had arrived. Sometimes people were late or needed to leave early, so whoever was in charge of facilitating the check-in was responsible for timing it to accommodate as many people as possible.

Normally, the director dictated the format that the check-in would follow for the day. It began with everyone sitting or standing in a circle and each member taking a turn to talk and move at the same time. The person talking/moving was expected to take the opportunity to stretch and warm up muscles, vocalize, and talk about himself or herself. When invited to speak with no specific instruction, people talked about how they were feeling, any difficulties they were having in life, or how their week was. More often than not, they disclosed information about their families, schools, work, and relationships. If the group had an upcoming performance scheduled and needed to rehearse specific sections of the performance, the director would also ask everyone to add comments on what parts of the performance they wanted to work on during rehearsal. For example, one might have been executing a series of neck rolls while saying, "I had a fight with my boyfriend this morning and I'm totally bummed out, and I think we need to work on the picture-posing section because it looked really bad at the last show." A check-in such as this served the dual purpose of (1) involving everyone in setting the agenda for the working process (such as working on the picture-posing section), and (2) accounting for any personal distractions (such as fights with the boyfriend). On other occasions, the director asked everyone to voice concerns or comments about a previous rehearsal, an artistic idea, or an interpersonal conflict between artists.

These directed check-ins in which people were given specific instructions about what to address, were done on top of regular check-ins to make sure everyone had an opportunity to talk. Moving/talking check-ins generally required active observation on the part of the people listening, since they were directed to copy or mirror the movement of the person talking. The interaction was set up so that everyone listened and watched each individual without themselves having to respond directly to what the speaker was saying. Check-ins helped establish and maintain intimate bonds between the members and prepared the performers' bodies for what was needed in rehearsal. *Laughter* required the performers to have the ability to move, talk, and improvise simultaneously; and checking in established the use of these skills—within an everyday exchange between members—as highly specialized and technical performance skills.

Initially, I found the process of checking in awkward, since people would often disclose very personal information. For the first two months, I would always choose to speak last and found myself trying to script something to say beforehand. I also found it unclear how much personal information I should disclose to a group of people with whom I was trying to establish a professional relationship. It was also difficult for me to ascertain how people reacted to personal divulgences, because the structure did not give people room to react to others' disclosures. For instance, someone might relate a story about a problem at home or work that she or he was trying to resolve. After the person was done talking, the focus would turn immediately to the next person who volunteered to lead the talking and/or moving, without any reference to the previous speaker's issues. After everyone had taken his or her turn, there would rarely be further discussion. Check-in offered a time to air one's feelings and thoughts as a way to "get them out of one's head," before further work was done during rehearsal.

Which Model of a Minority?

During check-ins, shared information deemed not discussable within a mainstream Vietnamese American community—a loose definition for anything labeled "not Club O' Noodles"—further established the rehearsal space as an alternative community within Vietnamese American and Asian American communities. During one of the check-ins, for example, Anh, a college student at the time, complained that her lab partner had given her a hard time earlier that morning for spending so much time rehearsing for an upcoming performance.[8] Anh's lab partner was Vietnamese American and told Anh she should be spending her time studying in order to get a good job after graduation, instead of wasting her time at rehearsal. Anh considered her lab partner's attitude typical of the mainstream Vietnamese American community that buys into model-minority stereotypes. Arguably, the lab partner was offering sound career advice, but Anh said she felt betrayed, because she (Anh) saw herself as someone who spent long hours working for the greater Vietnamese American community, which included her lab partner.

Anh's check-in revealed the irony of publicly representing one's own ethnic community while feeling alienated from it. She believed that her lab partner's aspiration to embody the model-minority stereotype undermined her efforts to challenge stereotypes and envision a new place for Vietnamese American history and culture in the United States. Anh found herself unable to craft a good argument against her lab partner's stated desire to get a good job after graduation. From an economic standpoint, the model minority is not necessarily a stereotype of limitations, so why does Anh view her lab partner's ambitions as shortsighted? Much of the critical literature on the model-minority stereotype focuses on the fact that the myth does not account for the segment of the Asian American population who are living in poverty and/or are working in economically exploitative situations. Both Anh and her lab partner are ostensibly middle-class Vietnamese American college students, so why does Anh characterize her lab partner's ambitions as an annoying case of self-internalized model-minority syndrome, but not see herself as a model minority? For Anh, to pursue art would make her downwardly mobile.

The model-minority stereotype offers up an image of racialized economic success determined by a formula of rationales for certain strategies and shortcuts. Working in the spirit of public-service announcements, education functions as the key to success for options in life. Thus, a university education and good grades are idealized as the most effective strategy for overcoming racial discrimination. High-profile cases of individual Asian American educational success (the valedictorian, the salutatorian, and so on) symbolize irrefutable evidence that Asian Americans are able to overcome all forms of adversity through personal achievement. These individualized acts are perceived as more effective than public protest (group complaint) at combating discrimination. The logic functions as a shortcut, because it rationalizes a methodology for economic-as-social success.

good grades → university education → good job → racial equality

The shortcut also requires the identification of disciplines both suitable and unsuitable for attaining objectively irrefutable (economic) success. Certainly, the humanities and performing arts (particularly, experimental performance art) fail to satisfy the logic of the shortcut at the point of "good job" and thus are subsequently excluded from model minorities' deracialized narrative of upward mobility.

Marginalizing artists is not limited to the Vietnamese American or the Asian American community, but is reflective of an endemic U.S. attitude that artistic labor is not "real work" or is, at most, supplementary culture. The model-minority approach amplifies this attitude, since it overdetermines Asian Americans as incipient capitalists. Since the immigration of Chinese laborers to the United States in the late nineteenth century, subsequent generations of Asian immigrants have been understood through the discourse of the "yellow peril" whose business acumen would undermine the social fabric of American life. Fear of the yellow peril centered around two beliefs: the first figures the Asian immigrant as inherently thrifty, unscrupulous, and overly concerned with money, thus the Asian worker holds unfair advantage over the average white American worker; the second figures the Asian immigrant through the lens of an Orientalist discourse that frames the Asian immigrant as a moribund victim of his own cultural excess generated by ancient and outdated cultural beliefs and practices.

This excess—tradition-bound despotism—functions as a persistent and imagined threat to U.S. perceptions of itself as a modern and politically progressive democratic society. Excess—naturalized as Asian cultural values —functions as an explanation for the absence of Asian Americans from contemporary American cultural life, the arts, and humanities. In the United States, art is quite often framed as an activity people engage in after the basics (one's economic well-being) are taken care of, and Asian immigrants are quite often thought of as fundamentally uninterested in art. Instead, Asian immigrants are framed as an economically successful population hampered by an inability to move beyond an obsession with money and thus unable to become fully realized and creative individuals. Boldness, creativity, and ingenuity—words often used to describe the American way of doing things—are replaced by hard work and self-sacrifice to describe the outcome of Asian labor. If American success is inspired by the creative spark, Asian success is framed as the result of laborious repetition.

Ahn's lab partner may have intended to offer sound career advice, not to reinscribe the model-minority stereotype; however, her expressed opinions about the path to success had that effect. The problem with the myth of the model minority is not that it is located in the moment of achieving success, but in how the stereotype equates success with naturalized political passivity and cultural distance. To make the fallacy of the stereotype visible requires taking the risk of incorporating economic failure into being Asian American. It *risks* a reading of failure, because the act of choosing to make visible the failure of the model-minority stereotype through non–model-minority behavior presumes involvement in endeavors marked as guaranteed economic failures. It therefore *requires* a willingness to be a failed capitalist in order to make visible the diverse realities of economic exploitation, underemployment, glass ceilings, and poverty experienced by Asian Americans.

Positive images of Asian Americans available via the model-minority stereotype help to rationalize a historically unstable right to be in the United States. Narratives of the successful immigrant who manages to achieve the markers of a middle-class lifestyle in spite of anti-immigrant or anti-Asian sentiment "prove" that Asian immigration is economically beneficial and not a burden on the American taxpayer (the Anglo-American worker). While Asian immigrants have no history of native land rights, slavery, or annexation, the projection of failure risks the public "right" to rationalize anti-immigrant and anti-Asian sentiment, because nineteenth-century U.S. labor history legislated the Asian immigrant as "returnable" labor. Asian American immigration history is one that is fragmented between the anti-Asian-immigrant legislation of the nineteenth and early twentieth centuries and the boom in Asian immigration post-1965. The conditions of post-1965 immigration from Asia were significantly different from those of nineteenth-century immigration; however, the rhetoric has not changed. Thus, legal American citizens of Asian descent are still viewed not only as *perpetual foreigners* but, more importantly, also as *returnable foreigners*.

The struggle to claim an identity as an artist—a career choice marked as a predetermined economic failure because it operates outside the parameters of the model-minority stereotype—proves difficult within a community that has much at stake in maintaining model-minority status as an economic argument for minimizing anti-immigrant and anti-Asian legislation and sentiments. The tolerance for racialized economic success is dependent upon many factors beyond the scope of the argument that I am trying to make here about the relationship between the Asian American artist and the model-minority stereotype. In returning to Anh, her check-in during rehearsal reveals that through her participation in Club O' Noodles she is allowed to claim an artistic identity without having to subscribe to a language of economic failure or success.

New Members

While moving through space, Anh related the conversation she had had with her lab partner. Instead of sympathizing or empathizing with her story, the rest of us mirrored her actions as she released her upper body into a forward bend. Rolling down her spine one vertebrae at a time, she let out a deep sigh as her head dangled inches from the floor. In response, we all sighed with her. Anh was a seasoned member of CON and looked forward to sharing her story with a group that would sigh with her in a kind of assumed agreement. It is true that as a group we were simply mirroring her movements, but in the context of her story, the group sigh sounded like a collective release of tension and frustration.

This pedagogical strategy of following and leading helped to establish a sense of community among the members of the group by dispersing the experience of leadership and technical skill. In Anh's case, following and leading served as an emotional outlet to vent frustration without turning her disclosure into a prolonged gripe fest. It would have been easy for everyone to chime in and relate their own stories about similar situations. Instead, Anh was able to disclose her frustration and receive both a visual and an aural response. She knew we were paying attention because we had to copy the precise placements of her body, the timing and quality of her movements, and the pitch and volume of her voice. In other words, we had to pay attention to more than just her story.

The dispersal of leadership also served another purpose: it disrupted traditional notions of how one could attain technical performance skills. Anh welcomed her moment in the spotlight during check-in and executed her turn with confidence. However, the fact that this was an acquired skill became apparent during the fourth rehearsal I attended, when one of the members brought two friends, Jenny and Linda. I arrived ten minutes late and everyone was already standing in a circle. Nguyen had asked each person to take turns leading a series of stretches—including Jenny and Lisa. It was apparent that both women were taken aback at how quickly Nguyen and the rest of the members integrated them into the group's activities. When Jenny's turn arrived, she scrunched up her face. She took some time to think and finally bent over to place her hands on the floor and pulled one leg behind herself to perform an awkward lunge. The position was difficult for her to maintain; she bounced up and down a few times, then quickly passed on the leadership role to the person next to her.

This pedagogical approach of giving everyone an opportunity to lead an exercise, whether she or he wanted to or knew how to, surprised the new members. They were not prepared to find themselves cast in a momentary leadership position. Jenny's experience typified how Club O' Noodles operated on the idea that anyone could participate in the collective effort of the group, regardless of previous experience. The organization was interested in creating opportunity based on interest, rather than creating exclusion based on evaluating skill level. Desire to be part of the company took precedence over preexisting performance skills. Members worked on the assumption that everyone would be able to develop specific skills as he or she continued working with the group. This does not mean that people did not have any acting, singing, or dance skills, but that the value placed on interest created a welcoming artistic atmosphere in which everyone could participate equally in a given activity. Instead of someone being assigned to teach a choreographed warm-up emphasizing technical precision, each individual led a short, improvised exercise so that both experienced and inexperienced members could successfully execute their own section of the warm-up. Even though it was difficult for the new members to take a leadership role within the first fifteen minutes of their arrival, they were able to draw upon movement vocabulary familiar to their own bodies.

Using an aesthetic of familiar movement vocabulary ("familiar" in the sense that a person can only lead what s/he can actually execute) to accommodate people with different skill levels is very much in the spirit of postmodern dance. Le, who had been a member of Club O' Noodles for about six months at the time that I met her, joined because she did not have to audition in order to be part of the group. She often said that this made the organization an inclusive and nurturing place. She kept emphasizing that "you don't have to have any talent." When I asked her what she meant by "talent," she explained that she did not think of herself as a particularly good actor, dancer, or singer, but she had a longstanding interest in theater. She thought other theater groups were elitist and would never have given her the opportunity to join them.

When Le first joined Club O' Noodles, she assumed that she would work backstage as part of the technical crew. Once she started attending rehearsals and workshops, Nguyen gave her a script and told her she was going to perform in a show scheduled for the following week. Her debut turned out to be a sold-out performance in a five-hundred-seat theater at California State University–Northridge. During the performance, Le and another performer, who joined the group around the same time, found themselves standing in the wings reading the script, trying to figure out what they were supposed to do next on stage.

The practice of throwing new members into the thick of things created a situation whereby new and interested members were assumed to have the potential to learn needed skills to perform on stage. The emphasis on inclusion via full immersion caused a certain amount of anxiety for new members. Like Jenny and her friend, I too felt a certain level of anxiety. My anxiety also included a struggle to understand what I was willing and unwilling to disclose during check-ins and other exercises that required talking about myself. Part of my anxiety had to do with the fact that I was a researcher who was also an ethnic outsider.

As a researcher, I was listening to people discuss personal issues about their sex lives, relationships, family conflicts, career anxieties, and a whole host of other issues. It was often overwhelming to imagine how I could possibly represent the contents of these interactions or whether I even wanted to. I did present myself as a researcher and talked about these anxieties during my check-ins, with the group as a whole, and with individual members. Even though I established this dialogue during the rehearsal process, there still remained the issue of writing about these experiences. Part of my dilemma stemmed from the fact that people volunteered personal information within a "safe" rehearsal space context established before my arrival. People volunteered information during the rehearsal process that I did not solicit, yet that information was relevant to my work because it often found its way onto the stage.

When Form Yields Unexpected Content

Even when I encountered moments of being "in the know," or actually possessing a modicum of authority on a subject in rehearsal, I continued to find myself in the role of the outsider for unexpected reasons. In chapter 4, I describe a contact improvisation workshop taught by Maura Nguyen Dono-hue. In the post-workshop discussion, one of the men, Phu (a pseudonym), admitted that he felt sexually aroused while dancing in the round-robin. I was unsure how to react in that moment, because in all of my previous experiences of learning and practicing contact improvisation, the topic of sexual arousal was a no-no. Post-jam discussions usually involved language emphasizing physical mechanics of weight, gravity, and support, or meta-physical experiences of trust, connection to particular individuals, being in one's body, or feeling the energy. These vocabularies avoid social narratives for the moving body such that the dancing body signifies a collection of forces described by scientific principles.

Phu's comments would most likely be interpreted as an artistic faux pas within traditional contact improvisational spaces. The unwritten rules sur-rounding contact improvisation imagine the practice as a democratic space where people of all skill levels can socially engage in a high-art dance form. It is a high-art dance form in the sense that it is supposed to be an experience of dancing with other "abstract bodies." To foreground sexual arousal disrupts this abstracted space by aligning the practice with commercial or popular dance forms that stage narratives of heteronormative gender roles and sexual desire. The appeal of contact improvisation lies in the ideological attempt to reclaim an entire range of bodily movement from clichés and metaphors that liken dance to romance and seduction.

I have to admit that I was disturbed by Phu's comment at the time, unsure if the other women were uncomfortable with his remarks. Within the context of traditional contact improvisational spaces, it would have been inappropriate, but we were in a different space; even then, my feminist self wanted to say something about Phu's comments during the post-workshop discussion. As a researcher, however, I could not tell Phu that his comments were inappropriate, because I was, in fact, observing how the group would react to his remarks. By the same token, I had already observed that the women in the group did not always voice their concerns during group meetings in the same way that the men did. I also wondered whether my discomfort arose from an entirely different place. Was my discomfort a result of my dance training and was my initial shock a result of an unacknowledged elitism? In my quest to unearth the transgressive nature of Club O' Noodles's work, did I come at it with a blind spot? Did my preconceived notion of what contact improvisation was supposed to mean get in the way?

I returned to traditional narratives of contact improvisation as an idealized practice that disentangles the moving body from heteronormative gender roles. And suddenly it dawned on me that such an ideal is not transgressive in a context where bodies are not seen through the lens of romance and sexual desire. In the case of Club O' Noodles, seeing Asian American bodies dancing with other Asian American bodies challenges the way in which Asian American bodies are not seen as sexual bodies within narratives of "normal" romantic relationships. Asian American male bodies are desexualized through narratives of asexual houseboys, laundry workers, and disembodied spiritual masters, and Asian American female bodies are hypersexualized through narratives of interracial prostitution. This representational setup excludes the possibility of Asian or Asian American couplings (regardless of sexual orientation). The issue of overpopulation (particularly the fixation on India and China) is an exception to the rule and couched as a generically Asian problem that can be fixed through scientific means. Asian sex is then a problem of uncontrollable reproduction and irresponsibility, much like the problem created by unneutered and unspayed pets.

While Phu's comments could be interpreted as conservative within the context of contact improvisation, they actually mirror the ideals set forth by contact improvisation and its ethos of being attuned to how one's body feels. In addition, Donohue's workshop occurred within another context: finding ways to reclaim the Asian American body. The social ideals and the practice of contact allowed the male dancer to acknowledge the presence of an Asian male body and reclaim Asian American male sexuality. This act of reclaiming the body still poses a conundrum for Asian American female bodies, since Phu's comment violated the unwritten rule about sexual neutrality. The premise of neutrality within contact improvisation is supposed to maintain a safe space for women to dance in a cogendered environment where heterosexual men are present. The hypersexualization of Orientalized Asian female bodies creates a situation in which Asian American women have a difficult time of reclaiming and representing Asian American female sexuality without being read as a reinscription of across-the-board availability.

The members viewed each other's company as a safe space to claim their sexual identity through frank disclosures during the check-in. Individuals would offer, "I had a really great orgasm this morning" as casually as "I have a cramp in my right rhomboid." At first, I was surprised at the matter-of-fact statements about people's sex lives during the rehearsal process, since it was not reflected in their performance work. Even though Club O' Noodles had a close relationship to Highways Performance Space, known locally as a queer space, Club O' Noodles was not marketed as a queer-identified company, nor did its performance work deal with sexual identity on a political level. Under the guidance of Hung Nguyen, whose solo work addressed explicitly queer Asian American identity, the rehearsal space became a neutralized, sex-positive space. What I mean by this is that whenever someone would disclose a narrative of sexual desire, it was not always couched in terms of a politicized sexual identity.

Although the assertion of sexuality is an important component of the rehearsal process, it does not find its way into the performance of *Laughter*. While there is a brief reference to an interracial relationship and homosexuality in *Laughter*, most of the references to sex are confined to parodies of the Asian female prostitute. In *Laughter*, Club O' Noodles deconstructed highly sexualized images of Asian female bodies, but did not offer an alternative representation of Asian American sexuality.

Performances like Michael Zia's *Exit the Dragon* (1994) attempt to recoup the desexualized Asian American male body by representing its opposite—the hyperhetero, hypersexualized Asian American male body. For Asian American women, reclaiming Asian female sexuality is trickier. Contrary to most popular filmic representations of Asian women as hypersexual prostitutes, Asian American female bodies are also desexualized as undesirable within white American beauty standards. More often than not, the off-screen stereotypes—small eyes, flat chests, and short legs—coupled with the model-minority image, operate to desexualize and pacify Asian American female bodies. Asian American girls and women may be overachievers in school, but they pose no real sexual threat. Under these circumstances, it makes sense that the attractive on-screen version of the Asian woman must fall under the rubric of prostitution. She is attractive for an Asian person, but must win the heart of the white hero through total submission or some inferred sexual perversion, both of which the liberated white woman does not need to assent to, because of her confidence, intelligence, and self-respect.[9]

Rehearsing Identity

If during stage performances of *Laughter*, Club O' Noodles was able to project a coherent representation of who or what constitutes Vietnamese American identity, this was not the case during rehearsals. Check-ins, and seemingly random workshop presentations, constituted the majority of the rehearsal process and did not specifically direct individuals to come up with Vietnamese American or Asian American material. References to Vietnamese or Asian American issues emerged out of individuals' engagement with the participatory nature of the improvisational structures that the group used, but these issues were in many ways quite different from the ones represented in the performance itself. If, in the public performance of *Laughter,* the group attempted to represent Vietnamese American identity via the legibility of mass popular culture, what emerged during the rehearsal process ranged from dissatisfaction with perceived Vietnamese American conservatism and a desire to constitute an alternative community, to a desire to luxuriate in the sensations of one's body.

This retreat into a body defined through the senses would prove temporary, for the kind of work Club O' Noodles aimed to create pulled the body back into dialogue with representation, thus exposing the political nature of the aesthetic structures con used in its rehearsal process. The interlude that follows, "The Amazing Chinese American Acrobat," as an embodied/performed investigation of the concepts of Club O' Noodles's work and process, takes as its subject the frictions between form and content. "The Amazing Chinese American Acrobat" is a written translation/reflection of a performed response to Club O' Noodles work. This "Asian American" performance piece is an account of the process of using choreography as a research methodology. The narrative goes through the paces of trying to work out the micropolitical relationship between form and content, the subject and object, and the self and the community, while simultaneously trying to make a decision about where to stand and what to wear. It is an exercise in working within the parameters of aesthetic and political choices offered by modern/postmodern dance and Asian American critique, as a way to understand where the blind spots are between the *doing of* (dance) and the *representing* (Asian American critique).

Interlude

THE AMAZING CHINESE AMERICAN ACROBAT
Choreography as Methodology

The Amazing Chinese American Acrobat suffers from a case of embarrassment and identification. Since she was six years old, she has longed to be a Chinese acrobat, after seeing on stage a young woman with shiny black hair and even shinier red pajamas twist herself into a knot while balancing on her hands sideways-up. The six-year-old thought to herself, "I could be like that." Not that she could really bend backwards until there was no space between her shoulders and the small of her lower back, but she thought to herself, "She (the woman on stage) is Chinese and therefore I (the six-year-old) who am also Chinese, or so the parents say, could be like that too." A moment of identification with the shiny black hair and even shinier red pajamas occurred one afternoon amidst enthusiastic oohs and aahs.

Twenty years later, the Amazing Chinese American Acrobat, who at this time has not yet quite committed to becoming the Amazing Chinese American Acrobat, once again sees a variety of Chinese acrobats who can juggle, spin, twist, balance, negotiate multiple objects and tasks deftly. This time, the Amazing Chinese American Acrobat finds herself responding with a subtle chill in her hair follicles, a slight increase in her heart rate, a marked rise in her skin's temperature. Yes, the acrobatic stunts are no less amazing, but somehow her response to her own identification with these Chinese acrobats is informed by an old memory that has taken a turn and made her nervous. She is all of a sudden hyperaware of all the other bodies sitting next to, in front of, and behind her and wonders if anyone else is experiencing a new discomfort, a feeling of embarrassment.

How to explain this new bodily sensation? The Amazing Chinese American Acrobat finds that she is not alone in her embarrassment. There are others blushing and who, like she, cannot resist the wonder of the spectacle. She finds a kindred spirit in theater historian James Moy (1993), who let it slip that he returned several times to Six Flags Great America outside of Chicago to watch the Chinese circus over and over again. He is critical of the circus, likening it to pornography and asserting that the festishization of Asian bodily virtuosity on stage functions as a denial of Asian American subjectivity through the disfigurement and denial of the Asian American body. Asian bodily virtuosity in the circus and in pornography signifies meaningless mastery over the manipulation of household objects. Chinese acrobats at the circus spin plates and balance ceramic pots on their heads. Spalding Gray's description of a live sex show in *Swimming to Cambodia* includes Thai women who shoot ping-pong balls and bananas out of their vaginas. Moy makes an astute observation that such mastery over household objects does not serve a utilitarian function other than unbelievable and exotic entertainment. In comparison to pornography, he points out that the Chinese acrobats at the circus offer the Anglo-American audience the most seemingly innocuous stereotype of Orientalized Chinese-ness and overall Asian-ness. He reads the costume and choreography of the Chinese acrobats as a collapsing of exotic Asian identities and an alleviation of U.S. fear of Asian virtuosity. I would argue that Moy's proposition functions in tandem with the model-minority stereotype in which Asian American economic and educational success (or virtuosity) are naturalized as unfair genetic propensities for math, science, and money.[1]

Of the costuming, he laments, "Wearing an assortment of curiously exotic ornamental costumes, which in more self-consciously avant-garde productions might be called postmodern, those on stage are marked as 'Chinese,' lest they be mistaken for some other ethnicity" (1993, 131). Of the choreography, he complains,

> Aside from the errant throw that sails far out of his reach, it seems the actor simply lowers his head at the last moment to allow the lime to bounce off his forehead—an appropriate gesture of self-effacement to deny complete virtuosity. In utopian America, complete mastery over everyday objects is at once denied and made Oriental,

mystified to yield a comfortable empire of the visual for middle-class America. (1993, 131)

But, what about the six-year-old aspiring Amazing Chinese American Acrobat and her parents who took her to such an event as a way of exposing her to "Chinese culture," so that she could get in touch with her roots, her background, ethnicity, history, and identity—the very Chinese-ness that embarrasses Moy?

This ideological gap between Moy's critique of the very performances that immigrant parents patronize and their desire to expose their children to their own cultural heritage signals the crisis that occurs between the space of multiculturalism and assimilation in the availability of American cultural offerings. The Chinese circus is real. It is as "authentic" as it gets. It is Chinese in the sense that it is performed by "real" Chinese bodies in China and abroad. Within middle-class Chinese American communities, a trip to see the Chinese acrobats functions along the same lines as Miss Chinatown pageants, Winter Blossom debutante balls, cultural shows, weekly lessons in folk dance, table tennis, brush painting, the all-important Chinese language class, and the ultimate: summer camp in Taiwan, mainland China, or Hong Kong. These camps are otherwise known as "The Love Boat," where participants can take part in activities in the "homeland" deemed proper and suitable for children of upwardly mobile, middle-class immigrant Chinese parents. Designed to provide second generations with an instant community, this social milieu operates as a preemptive strike against ethnic isolation and discrimination. At the same time, Moy's concerns are real and well-founded. The circus is a performance space with a tradition of spectacularizing specialty acts in accordance with narratives of national identity/character that draw upon easy-to-recognize visual and aural signifiers.

But how then do we account for the difference between Moy's assumed Anglo-American audience in Chicago whose exposure to such Chinese-ness takes place at an amusement park and my grandmother, a fifth-generation Chinese Malaysian living in Canada who stayed up all night to catch the Mandarin-language broadcast of a Chinese New Year variety show televised from Beijing that featured none other than Chinese acrobats. "Yu Tian, wake up, it looks like they have no bones."[2]

This essay, "The Amazing Chinese American Acrobat," is part III of a performance and research project I began in 1997. Over the years, it has sat on the shelf in boxes due to the formal demands of academic scholarship that quietly discourages too much self-reference and self-disclosure. "The Amazing Chinese American Acrobat" was originally a performance (of the same name) I created in an effort to find a new strategy for writing about the relationship between both aesthetic and political analyses of Asian American performances. Driving from one venue to another, seeing as many performances as I could possibly find, I found myself able to dissect other people's performances. "So-and-So's work debunks such-and-such stereotypes by reappropriating these kinds of stereotypes, in such-and-such a manner." In the end, I always found myself returning to the same question/conclusion: "Does the representation risk reinscribing the stereotype?" This approach to reading performance, no matter how sophisticated the twists and turns of my argument, was always haunted by the question "Is it a better representation?" I continually found myself back at square one, re-covering old territory in the methodological space that Asian American cultural criticism has been trying to get itself out of to move beyond the question of authenticity or accuracy.[3]

"The Amazing Chinese American Acrobat" is situated at this crossroad between Moy's critique and Chinese acrobats themselves. Moy dismisses the performances of the Chinese acrobats as a reactionary element within a particular Asian American sociopolitical agenda. The Chinese acrobats undermine what he considers self-consciously avant-garde performances by Asian American artists. But how do we account for the form and techniques of the circus? They obviously hold a certain amount of cultural value within communities that do not identify themselves as "Asian American," based on a conscious effort to build a pan-ethnic political coalition, not as culturally assimilated American citizens, but as Chinese immigrants. Considered "appropriate" family entertainment, unlike the majority of avant-garde performance art, the circus is something Chinese immigrant parents take children to see as an affirmation of cultural heritage.

Under these circumstances, it cannot be assumed—contrary to what Moy suggests—that self-consciously Asian American performance is somehow more representative or a superior representation of Asian Americans at large. In fact, charges of betrayal, airing dirty laundry, and just plain "weird" have been leveled at artists trying to walk the tightrope between community and individual self-expression. Just ask any self-identified avant-garde Asian American performance artists about the criteria they use to invite parents and other family members to their performances.

I gave myself the task of creating a self-consciously avant-garde Asian American performance to see what it would entail and to see if I could recuperate the form of the Chinese circus. Within the genre of contemporary Asian American performance art, Madame Butterfly stereotypes and the ilk have been made the cornerstones of parodies and satires in an effort to expose the ways in which they are Western fantasies about the Orient, and Oriental-ized female bodies in particular.[4] The Chinese acrobats pose a different set of issues, since Chinese bodies themselves produce both form and content. The female contortionist's solo is the highlight of the Chinese circus. She method-ically bends, twists, and places her limbs and torso into position: then, once she is ready, and only when she is ready, she turns her head to look directly at the audience, indicating, "Now you can applaud." It is this choreographed moment, this applause on demand, which never occurs before or after she is ready, that signals the agency of the performer and offers a possibility for my investigation in terms of understanding the gap between the circus's role as an empowering spectacle for Asian American children and its role as a source of racial embarrassment for James Moy. I was looking for a way to offer constructive advice to artists besides, "You are reiterating a stereotype, now try again."[5]

Lesson 1: The Politics of a First Work

Many Asian American performance artists are able to begin their careers as professional artists due to the perceived need for new talent. There is a high demand for new talent and new works, because the advent of multicultural programming has created new opportunities for artists of color. This search for new talent is often unconscious, since, in an effort to promote artistic diversity, it is frequently shaped by the need to find someone who has not performed at a particular venue or event in the last five years. The perceived lack of artists of color creates a situation in which Asian American per-formers must then "emerge" over and over again because student groups, alternative festivals, and venues willing to program experimental work by artists often have limited budgets that only allow them to program artists right before they become really famous and thus "too expensive."

As a result, Asian American performances that appear on stage are oftentimes either brand-new first works or first works that have already proven successful. First works tend to exorcise demons. They are also not necessarily an artist's first work at all, though they might be her or his first "Asian American work," and, as such, all previous history of the artist's work drops out of the picture. When people think of the 1990s Ping Chong, they think of his Asian trilogy and *Undesirable Elements,* but not his oeuvre of minimalist avant-garde works from the 1970s. *The Amazing Chinese American Acrobat* was my first (and, so far, only) Asian American work, in the sense that it was created with the intent of engaging with a body of Asian American cultural criticism. To my surprise, I managed to get more performance mileage out of this one work than any other dance I ever made. There was a niche for multicultural choreography that didn't seem to exist for "assimilated" abstractions.

Lesson 2: The Politically and Theoretically Watertight Performance

This journey into a first Asian American work generated a sense of urgency. This was the moment to address everything all at one time. Everything needed to be undone, reappropriated, and commented on from all angles. The performance needed to be watertight. It needed to anticipate all of the critiques that I knew I was capable of wielding when looking at someone else's work. This is where the divide, the bad feelings, the distrust between artists, critics, and scholars begin and often end. *Artists* are accused of not getting it quite right, *critics* are blamed for not getting it at all, or looking at the wrong thing, and *scholars* are accused of making it boring. Each retreats to her own corner feeling smug and secure that she knows what is best.

This scholarly trespass of going native, so to speak, and actually trying to choreograph at the intersection of theory and praxis, sheds light on the ironic situation in which Asian American artists and scholars do not always trust one another, even though they are battling the same forces of marginalization. Club O' Noodles, like many experimental performance ensembles, claims to value process over product; whereas, the critic presented with a process must still deal with a work-in-progress performance as a done deal. Works-in-progress are not without authorial intentions and representational repercussions.

It is passé to consider whether something is "authentic" or "better," but the criticisms of this practice, and the criticisms of the criticisms, have failed to produce new methods of critical analyses to analyze Asian American performance. At best, we have the established field of Asian American literary criticism and its "aesthetics of resistance," which has served as a springboard for finding a way to discuss other artistic disciplines and genres—film, theater, visual art, performance art, and dance.[6] Reading all cultural productions as texts within an aesthetics of resistance has become the preferred methodology, and the standard against which Asian American cultural production is compared to a political ideal.

For example, James Moy's critiques of David Henry Hwang's *M. Butterfly* and Philip Kan Gotanda's *Yankee Dawg You Die* situate both works as failures in fully recuperating Asian masculinity. *M. Butterfly* is based on a true story about the twenty-year love affair between a French diplomat named Bernard Bouriscot and his Chinese lover, whom he believed to be a woman. Bouriscot was arrested when French authorities discovered that the diplomat's lover was a spy. To add further intrigue, once the true identity of the Chinese spy was discovered, Bouriscot claimed that he had no idea that his lover was a man.

Hwang casts the story within a Madame Butterfly narrative, in which a French diplomat named Gallimard sees Song Ling Ling, a Chinese opera star, perform the aria from *Madama Butterfly* at a garden party in Shanghai. Unfamiliar with the convention of female impersonation in Chinese opera, Gallimard believes that Song is a woman; and, for the next twenty years, Song takes advantage of this mistake and continues to play the role of Madame Butterfly in order to extract information from Gallimard. Focusing on *M. Butterfly*, Moy argues that the character of Song Ling Ling only reinforces stereotypes of Asian men as effeminate and sexually suspect.[7]

Yankee Dawg You Die concentrates on the relationship between two Asian American actors as they struggle over what it means to be Asian American in Hollywood. Vincent Chin is the Hollywood veteran who, out of economic necessity, has passed as Chinese American (he is really Japanese American) in order to play Oriental stereotypes. Bradley Yamashita is a politically conscious Asian American actor who, at the beginning of the play, proclaims his refusal to play the kinds of "Oriental" roles that actors like Vincent, an actor of an older generation, portray. Moy is critical of *Yankee Dawg You Die* because the character Vincent is gay, which Moy equates with disfigurement and emasculation.

Michael Zia's *Exit the Dragon* reclaims Asian masculinity as undeniably heterosexual; however, it is also misogynist. In *Exit the Dragon*, three Asian American actors talk about the trials and tribulations of trying to break into Hollywood. After going through the litany of Asian male stereotypes, one of the actors longs for the day that he would get to "fuck white women." Alec Mapa's *I Remember Mapa* functions as an antidote to works like *Exit*; however, in the monologue about his adventures of navigating New York and Broadway as a queer Filipino man, women are still completely left out of the picture.

These ways of comparing *M. Butterfly*, *Exit the Dragon*, and *I Remember Mapa* still emanate from the question, "Is the work a better, or more accurate, representation?" Although the primary concern of the comparison is situated around how different critics and artists read and construct Asian and Asian American masculinity, the project can easily ignore aesthetics and turn into something that champions works that can demonstrate an appropriate ratio of aesthetics to political awareness. Works that lean toward experiments with aesthetic form as their primary concern are considered "different," "a new direction," "a challenge"—but never a foundation. Missing from textual analysis that focuses on the political efficacy of narrative content is attention to the ways in which artists are or are not making aesthetic innovations. In this case, *M. Butterfly* happens to be the performance that deploys aesthetic elements not entirely contained in the playscript. Hwang's use of the Chinese opera and Kabuki in the play offers another mode of interpretive entry into *M. Butterfly*, whereas the transcription of Alec Mapa's *I Remember Mapa* is legible in text as a comic monologue. However, Mapa's monologue is funnier if one is familiar with *M. Butterfly*, Hwang's deployment of the *kurago*, and Mapa's self-described covert attempts as a *kurago* to upstage the star of *M. Butterfly*, B. D. Wong. My point here is not to vilify the critic, but to keep in sight the fact that methodology informs interpretation.

Lesson 3: Choreographic Decisions and the Differences between Art and "Art"

MOVEMENT VOCABULARY

The Amazing Chinese American Acrobat cites the Chinese acrobat's repertoire; but how to do it given the framework provided by Moy's critique? Simply inverting the stereotype by re-producing tricks within a different narrative context would not suffice: it would fall under the rubric of reinscription, since the trick is still there. Yet, it is crucial to imagine the physicality of the acrobat as a strong, agile, athletic body. Aside from the recent appearances of Lucy Liu, Michelle Yeoh, and Michelle Kwan in the mainstream media, the idea of seeing the Asian female body as physically adept and not just physically desirable is largely absent in the United States. The popularity of Lucy Liu and Michelle Yeoh as kick-ass action s/heroes and Michelle Kwan as figure skater extraordinaire relies on the hyperfeminized associations between practice and gender. Marital arts are associated with the "feminized" East. Figure skating—with its dual role as a subjectively judged competitive sport (some other sports have strictly objective guidelines governing the measurement of speed, distance jumped, or tasks completed) and a competition with glitzy costumes, music, and choreography—looks too much like frictionless dancing, that other activity also marked as feminine and gay.

I chose to use the Chinese acrobat's transitional vocabulary; in other words, the gestures and movements the acrobat and her assistants use to indicate the beginning and end of a spectacular moment. A solo performer might be flanked by assistants whose job it is to direct the audience's attention to the "star." The precision of the execution and the timing of the gestures are crucial to establishing how audiences can be trained to respond appropriately to what they see. "Audiences are smarter than that," or so I have been told. But are they? Broadway musicals such as *Miss Saigon* and the revival of *Flower Drum Song* have cashed in as "Asian American" performances, based on their supposedly authentic representations of Vietnamese and Chinese Americans.

COSTUMES

The costumes proved more difficult to think through. To wear the shiny pajamas would play into the stereotype, yet the recognizability of a familiarly exotic costume is part of its visual appeal. At the same time, it is a bona fide, authentic costume. In her closet, my mother had one of those satin pink-and-green numbers with a floral appliqué sewn on the chest. It was left over from the days when she danced in Frank Que's Chinese folk-dance troupe in the 1970s and 1980s. When I was a child, my mother's dancing seemed like a natural extension of our family's Chinese-ness, as if it were a diasporic lowest common denominator; or, from my ten-year-old point of view, a kind of ethnic purgatory. My father, always the firm believer that China would eventually assert its place in the global economy, decided early on that Mandarin would become his family's lingua franca so that his children would have a leg up when it came time to look for a job. This was something I only realized as an adult when I discovered that close relatives who grew up in the "homeland" didn't speak the same "useful" Chinese that I did. Bilingualism in this case was not so much a matter of transmitting Chinese cultural values or preserving cultural heritage, but of conscientiously attempting to assimilate into a middle-class Chinese American-ness informed by the rise of Monterey Park—the new, suburban, Mandarin-speaking Chinatown—rather than into the working-class, Cantonese-speaking old Chinatown.

As I mentioned earlier, accompanying my mother to her rehearsals was like an ethnic purgatory—"purgatory" in the sense that national differences were elided in the service of performing a Chinese-ness that, on one hand, had everything to do with everyday life. Each time I saw my mother in full stage makeup and costume, I was rendered speechless by her fur-trimmed tunics, rhinestone earrings, blue eye-shadow, and fan—gold on one side, silver on the other. She was a woman transformed—otherworldly and exotic. No longer was she the woman who waited for me in a sweltering car with my baby brother in the back seat while I attended my piano lesson. On stage and backstage, she became a public figure, a cultural ambassador, a living embodiment of five thousand years of Chinese history.

My younger sister refused to let me borrow her competition *wu shu* silks, suspecting that I was probably going to be doing something strange in them.[8] The costume posed a dilemma. To wear an authentic costume would risk reiterating the stereotype, since it smacked of Chinatown tourism, another source of embarrassment and identification. Chinatown is that place where middle-class Chinese Americans go for dinner but would not be caught dead living in, knowing full well that non-Asian tourists think one's bodily presence alone is part of a charmingly exotic cultural experience. In addition, wearing the costume in a self-consciously avant-garde context could be read as making fun of something taken very seriously in Chinese dance and martial arts communities. Even if tourists buy those $29.99 shiny red pajamas for their little girls to wear on Halloween, so did our Huntington Beach Chinese School dance teacher, with her degree in Chinese folk dance from a Taiwanese university. She bought them for us to wear at our annual Chinese New Year Culture Show and Picnic. In the end, my mother gave me her pink-and-green satin costume, which had been sitting in the back of her closet for the last twenty years. It turned out to be about three sizes too small for me, so instead of directly wearing it, I wore it Velcroed to the front of my T-shirt and sweatpants. My sister was right.

Creating a Performative Autoethnography

Not until 1997 did the Amazing Chinese American Acrobat finally commit to her new role, while attending rehearsals and performances of Club O' Noodles's *Laughter from the Children of War* and *Stories from a Nail Salon*. She needed to sort out what quickly became an accidental ethnography, once observing rehearsal transformed into full-blown "fieldwork," or what Visweswaran (1994) and Kondo (1997) call "homework." Key members of Club O' Noodles realized the acrobat/ethnographer had some useful skills and put her to work assisting with grant writing, proofreading, standing in for absentee performers during rehearsals, and sometimes performing.

Yes, the Amazing Chinese American Acrobat is this ethnographer's alter ego, dreamed up to co-choreograph on paper a performative autoethnography—a methodology concerned with representing the process of creating performances and performing (the doing of) ethnographic research. Here, the acrobat moves behind the camera, in front of the camera, on stage with other dancing bodies, on a panel with other talking heads, and alone in front of the computer.

She is never completely alone and is always able to find other co-conspirators. At the 2001 annual meeting of the Association for Asian American Studies, four panels on Asian American theater and dance appeared on the program. Performance had finally made it into the mainstream of Asian American studies. Not only did it mean Asian American performance studies was finally taken seriously as a topic of scholarly inquiry, but it also meant that there were finally enough people writing about performance such that one could see different theoretical and methodological approaches emerging. The panel "Performing Cultural Interventions: Community and Asian American Theater" generated a series of questions regarding the relationship between the researcher and research subject when the boundaries of both are blurred—something that made the Amazing Chinese American Acrobat sit up in her seat.[9]

Though not the topic of the panel, these questions emerged during the course of the question-and-answer session. The three panelists presented work categorized as "community theater," which included experimental performance events, professional organizations, and theater venues. All the presenters worked as performers within their respective organizations, but each panelist presented him- or herself as a researcher presenting research on an organization and not an artist representing an organization.

Ironically, all of the presenters could be considered living embodiments of the ideal Asian Americanist—the scholar who is at once artist and activist —but none of the panelists presented their research from the point of view of the scholar/artist. This is what my performative autoethnography attempts to address. Each presenter's dual role as researcher and subject of his or her own research was evident by way of embarrassed disclaimers when the scholar/performer's body showed up in video clips during the presentations. This attempt to mask the fact that one's information was procured through avenues other than solitary library study and properly distanced participation/observation was an unexpected denial in a field (Asian American studies) that perceives itself as the proponent of the ideal academic citizen: the scholar/artist/activist. So, why this embarrassment? Is it the performer's fear of looking bad on video or the scholar's fear of "going native" on paper? This question is not meant to be simplistic, but points toward the unstable place of dance and theater as subjects of scholarly inquiry in the academy.

Unlike other researchers, the scholar/artist is an idealized norm rather than the exception in dance studies. (Few expect art historians to exhibit artwork in juried shows.) This practice may sound like the ultimate integration of theory and practice, but such practices do not usually emerge out of a radical vision of interdisciplinary pedagogy and research. More often, it is a matter of economics, which demands jack-of-all-trades faculty in small dance departments and demands artists to find other ways to support themselves than art-making. Since the late 1980s, dance scholars trying to push the topic of dance further into the center of the academy, while reclaiming its sudden popularity among literary scholars, have done so under the premise that competency in the dance technique related to one's research topic would provide an important leg up in producing cutting-edge scholarship—thus reiterating the practice of equating proficiency in dance technique with proficiency in dance scholarship. I am not advocating that proficiency in technique does not inform scholarship or that technique cannot be a form of research, but what I am alluding to is the danger that such an assumption can discount the specificities of dance scholarship as a field with its own history, methodologies, and theoretical frameworks.

There is also another division—between the idea of dance *history* and the idea of dance *anthropology*—that I am trying to challenge. Unsaid but understood within the field is the premise that historical and anthropological methodologies mark racial and ethnic categories, such that Joann Kealiinohomoku's essay, "Ballet as Ethnic Dance" (1983), remains a radical anomaly. Cynthia Novack's *Sharing the Dance* (1990) and Jennifer Fisher's *Nutcracker Nation* (2003) are two notable exceptions in that both are ethnographic studies of white theatrical dance, and the "ethnographic-ness" of each study is central to the identity of the writing. Novack sees contact improvisation as more like folk dance than concert dance, and thus as an obvious subject of anthropological inquiry. Kealiinohomoku's concern regarding ballet and its ethnicity does not have so much to do with ballet itself as with the recognition that ballet exists within a cultural context. Fisher's book-length study of regionally produced *Nutcracker*s answers Kealiinohomoku's call. Neither of the latter two ethnographies claims self-reflexivity on the part of the ethnographer, nor does either deploy radical anthropological methods. Curiously, both read differently from traditional ethnographies in that they focus on the practices and thus lack the exoticizing tendencies typical of traditional ethnographies in which descriptions of the dance form are accompanied by accounts of what the subjects eat and how they live. There is an ease with which Kealiinohomoku, Novack, and Fisher are able to write as "native" anthropologists.

I attribute this ease to contact improvisation's and ballet's solid situations within dance history. These forms are well documented within the discipline of dance history, so using anthropological methods signals a radical move that remains marginal or particular within the larger context of history. In other words, Fisher's ethnographic account is but one in a large corpus of writing about nineteenth-century story ballets. Its ideal reader is the balleto-mane who already attends *The Nutcracker* every year. For the non-Western, non-white body, the issue of methodology is trickier because ethnography is not viewed as an intervention but as an expectation. One reason that comes to mind as to why non-Western practices are subject to anthropological research is the perception that certain practices are irreproducible due to geographical distance from the center of a Western reading/viewing audience or culturally specific spontaneity. The issue of irreproducibility is really a distraction from the larger problem: the lack of official (written) histories.

Asian American performance suffers from the double lack of both written and oral histories.[10] For this reason, artist/scholars and scholar/artists like the three panelists are going out into the field, or have come in from the field, to make this history evident as a form of activism. This is particularly the case if one contextualizes performance within Asian American studies as a tradition of resisting or transforming Eurocentric canons of history, literature, and culture. The three panelists did not name their research methods as "ethnographic," nor did they self-identify as "native" ethnographers, even though their research was a result of their insider status within the organizations they wrote about. I frame their subject position as "native ethnographers" as a rhetorical move because Dan Bacalzo brought up the issue of his own subject position during the post-panel discussion.[11]

Fearing that readers might read his work as confessional at best, or the airing of a community's dirty laundry at worst, Bacalzo was concerned with how one chooses the limits of what one can write about without betraying the trust of friends and collaborators. He admitted to making the active decision not to discuss his own performance work, even though administrative work directly affected the form and content of the entire performance event that was the subject of this lecture. I believe such a confession signals a crisis in Asian American cultural critique, whereby the necessity of supporting and claiming the existence of one's community collides with the practice of offering honest or useful criticism. This is a topic discussed in hushed voices in hallways at conferences and in frustrated telephone conversations, and is in and of itself a form of dirty laundry. In his presentation on the New York–

based performance ensemble Peeling the Banana, Bacalzo purposefully left out an analysis of his own work. He carefully chose sections of other performers' work to illustrate Peeling's self-defined goals. And maybe the central question is, "To what extent are the organization's goals also those of the scholar/artist?"

This interlude—an account of a conscious attempt to enact a theory into practice, find the political in an aesthetic, use the content of a form, and merge the high and low—acts as a bridge between writing about the choreography of finished work and writing about choreography as it is made. The following chapter is also an ethnographic account of Club O' Noodles and its rehearsal process, with a return to the idea of rehearsing identity; however, the collective's attempt to better articulate a group identity was informed by market pressures of needing to revamp promotional material while in the midst of creating new work. If, in the previous chapters, Club O' Noodles appeared to espouse an egalitarian and individual approach to self-expression in the interest of inclusiveness, the next chapter demonstrates the limits to the collective approach.

The next chapter addresses the unsaid but understood distance and proximity of Club O' Noodles to a larger pan—Asian American performance scene. In trying to craft specific Vietnamese subjectivities, the group drew upon the resources of the greater Asian American performance community in Los Angeles to provide workshops and guidance to achieve particular artistic as well as political goals. The following narrative investigates the negotiations of racial sameness and ethnic difference that appear fluid yet are clearly defined.

4

MAPPING MEMBERSHIP
Class, Ethnicity, and the Making of
Stories from a Nail Salon

Outing the Ethnic Other

I traveled with Club O' Noodles to their performances at schools, museums, and theaters up and down the coast of California. At first my main responsibility was to run the video camera at each show; over time, I was assigned an increasing number of jobs. One of the first tasks involved facilitating postshow discussions. I would go out on stage after the curtain call and encourage people to stay after the show for discussion. This allowed the cast a few extra minutes to change out of sweaty costumes and regroup before returning to the stage to talk to the audience. Eventually I became an understudy, and by the time Club O' Noodles premiered *Stories from a Nail Salon*, I contributed material to its work.

After facilitating my second post-show discussion, I realized that some people in the audience assumed that I was Vietnamese American. There was the elderly white woman who approached me after a show to tell me how wonderful it was that "my people" could overcome such great hardship and succeed in America, as well as the white museum employee who flagged me down to enlist my help in handing out the beautifully thin sheets of intricately patterned "Vietnamese paper" to all the children attending the arts festival that Club O' Noodles had performed in.

Of course, I took delight in telling the well-meaning white woman that I was not Vietnamese, nor was I in the performance that she had just seen. And, of course, I told the museum employee that perhaps all the Chinese American parents in attendance might find it inappropriate for someone to give Chinese funerary money to children. Responses to my clarifications of these and other misreadings ranged from not seeming to notice, substituting some other Asian ethnicity for Vietnamese in the rest of their comments, confused sputtering ("but, I thought . . ."), or simply staring for a moment, then walking away. In many ways, these kinds of reactions were familiar insomuch as I, like many Asian Americans, have experienced them in every-day situations at school, work, the grocery store, the bank, and on the street.

What I did not expect was the dilemma of mistaken identity posed by Asian American audiences, and Vietnamese American audiences in particu-lar. The case of mistaken or assumed identity isn't uncommon in everyday life—going about one's business in ethnic shopping centers and business districts. A simple, "Sorry I don't speak ——," will usually suffice, and the transaction continues without missing a beat. In everyday life, ethnic passing might have benefits, such as the "co-ethnic discount" or the "special menu." In such situations, a number of little things are to be gained by not making too much of a point about difference. This kind of ethnic misidentification takes on an entirely different meaning when the geographic space and tem-porality of everyday life become reframed as one's field site.

One evening after a show, I was standing in the theater next to Anh. We were getting ready to go backstage to clean up and return to the hotel where we were staying, when a large contingent of her extended family came over to surprise her with a big bouquet of flowers. Most of the people in the audience had already left, but a good number of people were still milling about, greeting friends, and waiting for a chance to talk to the performers. Anh had not seen her relatives in a long time and was busy exchanging hugs. As Anh moved deeper into the circle of people around her, I stepped back from the group to give them room to talk to Anh. As I did this, a middle-aged Vietnamese American man walked over to me. He was alone and I could tell that he had been waiting for a chance to talk to one of the per-formers and had wanted to talk to Anh (who played several of the major parts in the performance), before she suddenly disappeared into a sea of relatives. As the group around Anh grew louder, it was clear that it would be a while before Anh would be available for comment. So the man turned his attention to me, exclaiming, "It's so wonderful to see *you*—the younger generation of Vietnamese Americans—take on such difficult and important issues in the performance that *we* [in reference to himself] the older genera-tion, don't talk about."

I was clearly included in this collective "you" and the stakes seemed much higher, as evidenced by my awkward sputtering as I tried to explain that I was, in fact, not Vietnamese. Dance history is already full of stories about American women whose self-fashioned personas include narratives of mistaken identity: although Ruth St. Denis and Martha Graham, in their quests to define a new American dance, never claimed to be the exotic in their approximations of the other, Esther Luella Sherman transformed herself from a white, Midwestern woman into Ragini Devi, "a girl of Kashmir, a high-caste Brahmin who had spent much of her childhood in the secret sanctuaries of India and Tibet."[1] As Marta Savigliano observes in her study of tango tourism in Argentina, reporting momentary proximity to native practitioners and their blessings can yield a financially lucrative, status-building dance biography.[2] Savigliano describes a system in which it is considered good business practice for local dance teachers in Argentina to flatter the right American and European dance tourists on their techniques or feel for the dance. Teachers even hint that certain students may actually be able to pass for local dancers.

In general, the cross-ethnic casting of Asian American performers is a common practice in Asian American performance, which might be noticed but not necessarily commented upon. Asian American critics may decry the ubiquitous use of Filipino bodies in the global circulation of *Miss Saigon*, or debate whether the casting of a Filipino or Taiwanese American actor in the role of The Engineer is an improvement over Jonathan Pryce in yellowface.[3] For the general public, the concern over the absence of Vietnamese actors in *Miss Saigon* is a matter of splitting hairs. In 2000, almost a decade after *Miss Saigon* made its debut in London, Phong Truong was one of the first Vietnamese American actors cast in an adult role.

Given the politics of Club O' Noodles's self-defined Vietnamese American identity and its critique of *Miss Saigon*'s casting practices in *Laughter,* I found such ethnic passing, or at least the failure to disclose, a breach of contract. Vietnamese American reactions to the work included the recognition of collective memories. Artistically, the experimental structure of the performance worked because of the unspoken but assumed contract in which both Club O' Noodles and Vietnamese American audiences (who recognized themselves in the performances) could claim mutual ownership over the stories told in the performances. The stakes were different with non–Vietnamese American audiences and particularly with non–Asian American audiences. There were times when, outing myself to white audience members, I fantasized that somehow revealing my "true" identity would, in that moment of awkward sputtering, destabilize visual conflations of race, ethnicity, and nationality.

What, then, would this mean in terms of writing an ethnographic representation of Club O' Noodles's work? Is there a difference between the politics of performing a character on stage—when the work of performing is visible but not recognized—and writing ethnography? I am always working from a place of discomfort caused by reading critiques of ethnography and imagining my own subject position and participation in the representation of others. In the back of my mind are Edward Said's critiques of the very methodology I am using. In "Representing the Colonized: Anthropology's Interlocutors" (1989), Said questions whether recent anthropological efforts have moved beyond the project of Western imperialism. He situates the discipline of anthropology within what he calls "a crisis in representation" (205). This crisis is not exclusive to anthropology, but applies to all aspects of literary theory, humanities, and social sciences. The methods and motives used to produce narratives about other cultures are coming under increasing scrutiny, and Said points to the gaps between anthropologists' self-reflexive intentions and what they actually produce. He bases his argument on the fact that anthropology and ethnographic writing were methodologies created not only for the purpose of scholarly curiosity, but also as part of administering foreign policy (214–15). Western imperialism, he asserts, entails the creation of otherness and difference in order to establish authority. Said leaves off with the possibility for anthropology to be something other than itself by looking at "exile, immigration, and the crossing of boundaries" as potential ways to struggle against its imperialist tendencies (225).

Said's proposal for an anthropology that would resist reinscribing otherness into its narratives comes at the end of a list of sophisticated but failed anthropological projects by well-meaning writers. These failures, he argues, are based on anthropologists' dismissal of "native" anthropologists and their work. Though Said does not elaborate on the role of the native anthropologist, he suggests that the native anthropologist serves as "adversarial resistance to the discipline and the praxis of anthropology" (219–20). He also observes that the problem is not a lack of native anthropologists, but that anthropologists either ignore contributions made by native scholars or treat native anthropology as ethnographic data in need of interpretation. Herein lies the researcher's need to assert authority in order to write about a topic and to write in a manner that reveals the inherent interpretive process of writing about someone else's work.

Said's critique of anthropology and ethnographic writing points not only at a disciplinary crisis within anthropology, but to the very crisis of representation. In problematizing the representation of the other, he problematizes authority itself. Unequal power relationships between Western academics and their subjects/objects of study are translated by the authority of the anthropologist into categorical and objectified difference and otherness. The native anthropologist is not exempt from perpetuating such a crisis of representation. In fact the native is doubly subjected by a history of being represented and being held to the standards of anthropological critique. It is the native who understands full well the limits of anthropology. The dynamics of misrepresentation have driven the discipline of Asian American studies, making Asian Americanists attuned to perceived misrepresentations by fellow Asian Americans.

José Limón (1994) writes as a native who is painfully aware of his class privilege, marked by his college education and profession as a professor and anthropologist. It is this privilege that allows him to write about his own community, one of which he is no longer a part. Critiques of anthropological discourse look toward authentic voices, but does it allow for the practice of native self-representation, since attaining the tools and the time to write self-representative ethnographies forces the native to be categorized as an "outsider"? Methodologies for gathering research data and writing are also cast as inherently colonizing practices, so that native self-representation is impossible when scrutinized under the same critiques of traditional anthropology. Limón recognizes the contradictions of his subject position. He harbors what Anna Scott (1997) would call "proprietary instincts" for Mexican-American culture in south Texas while remaining nervous about the politics of his claim to authority. He is in a place where he has the tools to write in opposition to academically sanctioned misrepresentations and stereotypes about Mexican-American bodies and culture. When he attempts to criticize Anglo claims about the essential lower-class Mexican character as lascivious, lewd, and immoral, he faces his own self-doubt about how his work will be read. Limón writes:

Why do my people dance? But also, by what right does a working-class/Mexican-descent anthropologist dare approach the sordid edges of such a stereotype? ... In the 1970s I danced and drank (yet the other stereotype) with the continuing poor, uneducated and mixed-bloods of south Texas, but, unlike Walker's ancestors, I offer another cultural poetics, one, no doubt, also carrying its own repressions and contradictions, like those of my ethnographic precursors. (155)

In *Fictions of Feminist Ethnography* (1994), Kamala Visweswaran's interrogation of her identity as a first-world, mixed-race, Indian American anthropologist deconstructs practices of othering and identification within traditional anthropology, feminist anthropology, and identifying ethnography. She considers time spent living with her grandmother and cousins in Madras, India, as part of her fieldwork. Writing about her family, particularly her grandmother, would appear to be native anthropology. In the chapter, "Sari Stories," Visweswaran demonstrates how she negotiated her identity with other Indian women through the buying and wearing of saris. She writes, "Various concerned mamis, surprised and delighted with how 'Indian' I looked, determinedly gave me saris at all possible moments. ... Even distant members of the family commented on how much I looked like my grandmother" (166–67). It is in these moments of physical likeness and being with one's own blood relations that the wide gaps in age, class, and cultural differences that lead to misunderstandings, even in native ethnographies, are revealed.

Limón writes of a similar subject position and refers to his own trespasses as "less observation, more participation" (177). Writing as a native who grew up in a working-class Mexican American community, and having danced the same polkas during his youth, Limón is also painfully aware that his college education and profession mark him as an outsider. He relates a story that betrays his own class consciousness and his fear of actually being mistaken for one of his informants:

We drive our cars down to the big K-Mart parking lot down the street. As we spread the food, I tell them my Chicano K-Mart joke: What are the first words in English that a Chicano kid learns? "Attention K-Mart shoppers, we have a special on Aisle Four." They don't get it. I gnaw on a bone and ponder the complexities of the new bilingual joke. My wealthy lawyer friend likes it a lot. So do I. We're virtually alone on the K-Mart lot. Halfway through the bucket, my car next to Tony's, it occurs to me that we might look like a dope deal in progress to some passing police cruiser. Oh Lord. I wonder if *la rata* and/or Tony are carrying stuff as they sometimes do? Cold fear. *San Antonio Light* headlines: UTSA Prof. Deals Dope. Dissertation not Done. Prof. Done Gone. Will my university benefits cover a good lawyer? Small fat chance. Chicken. Gnawing fear. . . . I mentally rehearse my routine: Oh no, officer, You see, here's my faculty I.D. I have a Ph.D. . . . almost. Fat small chance. I wonder if there's a library in Huntsville. Will they let me out for the defense? (152)

His self-deprecatory Chicano joke clearly marks his current class privilege, provided by his education, his ability to speak English, and his financial power, which allows him to shop elsewhere—at middle-class stores, not K-Mart. Being poor is only funny in retrospect. Limón has caught himself telling an unfunny and classist joke in a situation in which poverty is real. The joke is also racist and no longer funny once Limón realizes that the police would not "see" his education and his fieldwork on a body that is racially and thus socially indistinguishable from that of his "informants."

Visweswaran uses failure as a framework for her ethnography. This is not to say that her project is a failure, but that she uses events of failure (the failed interview, misunderstandings, disregarded texts) as a basis for her ethnography. She is wary of the difficult position that she is in, since she wants to write a feminist ethnography from the point of view of a second-generation Indian American woman who writes about Indian women. She recognizes that the discipline that she is writing within has not yet addressed a set of issues brought forth by her circumstances. Her critique is not only a critique of ethnography, but also a meditation on whether or not there can actually be a feminist ethnography. Visweswaran accuses male ethnographers of focusing on the practice of identifying otherness and difference, while women ethnographers fall into the trap of assuming similarity with their female subjects.

It is at this point that the voice of the native comes in. From the stand-

point of Western academic practices, both Limón and Visweswaran embody
the subject position of the studied, simultaneously being and not being the
subject as object. In addition to problematizing the native anthropologist,
Visweswaran questions the validity of the separations between ethnography,
autobiography, and fiction. She does this to demonstrate how the gendering
of anthropology marginalizes ethnographies written by women anthropologists. "Feminist ethnographies" are marginalized as being subjective, confessional, and novelistic instead of critically self-reflexive. She uses the examples
of Zora Neale Hurston and Ella Deloria, two women of color whose works
she claims are read as novels instead of self-consciously experimental ethnographies that challenge not just the form but also the power relationships
inherent in ethnographic writing.

Visweswaran's critique of experimental ethnographies championed by
anthropologists such as James Clifford calls attention to the fact that experimental anthropology is recognized only when there is still a clear distinction
between the researcher and the subject. She writes,

> I am not surprised that no inclusion of work done in ethnic studies
> or so-called indigenous anthropology is made in experimental eth-
> nography, but I am dismayed. This, despite the fact that these writ-
> ings explicitly challenge the authority of representations . . . of them-
> selves. Self writing about like selves has thus far not been on the
> agenda of experimental ethnography. To accept "native" authority *is*
> to give up the game.
>
> If we have learned anything about anthropology's encounter
> with colonialism, the question is not really whether anthropologists
> can represent people better, but whether we can be accountable to
> people's own struggles for self-representation and self-determina-
> tion. (31–2; emphasis in original)

Visweswaran views experimental ethnography as a failed strategy because
the crisis of representation remains when ethnography is narrowly defined.
In this regard, she advocates taking Said's critique a step further in terms of
laying out how to chip away at the borders of anthropological canons: "When
the 'other' drops out of anthropology, becomes subject, participant, and *sole*

author, not 'object' then, in Kevin Dwyer's words, we will have established a 'hermeneutics of vulnerability' and an 'anthropology which calls itself into question' " (32; emphasis in original).

Within autobiography, the subject/object is also the authorial voice. When autobiography is included in the consideration of what can be constituted as an anthropological text, the overlap between writer as authority and writer as subject calls into question the relationship between subjectivity and agency. For an anthropologist to critique autobiography, the writer must address questions of genre and the subject/author's self-representational practices. According to Visweswaren, including autobiography is a way for anthropology to engage with a subject without reproducing representations based solely on otherness.

Working with Club O' Noodles required my body to remain present, and, even as I tried to recede to the sidelines as a disembodied observer, I was always called into the circle whenever I looked a little too comfortable. If Club O' Noodles had allowed me to remain comfortably distanced from the action, I could have retreated to locating myself as an Asian American workshop participant writing about Asian American performance workshops. But the process called forth my subject position as a Chinese American woman writing about and performing with a Vietnamese American performance ensemble—and this practice points toward a politics of racial and ethnic identifications/disidentifications of doing Asian American performance ethnography.

Draw Who You Are

After a month in the field, Nguyen announced to the group that he had invited Steve (a pseudonym) to help facilitate Club O' Noodles's next meeting. Nguyen felt it was time for Club O' Noodles to assess where the company was headed both administratively and artistically. The plan was to hold a series of meetings in which the company would write a new mission statement, to be used for grant proposals and press releases. The mission statement would also serve to define CON's niche in the performance art world. Trained in leadership counseling, Steve was a Japanese American teacher who taught conflict resolution and multicultural education in a large public school district in Southern California. From the researcher's point of view. I thought this was going to be an ethnographic gold mine. I could witness how individual members viewed themselves as well as the organization. More importantly, I was going to have the opportunity to listen in on how Club O' Noodles planned to represent and market itself to potential presenters and audiences.

For a moment, I thought my ethnographic anxieties regarding the power relationships between researcher and researched would subside, because I was no longer the nosy researcher asking intrusive questions relevant only to my research project. Instead of my asking questions, the group had invited someone else—a trusted person familiar with the organization—to facilitate the discussion about each individual's role within Club O' Noodles. Questions included. "What do individual members want from their participation in the group?" and "What direction do individual members want the organization to take?" In addition, the workshop leader was an ethnic outsider, yet he was invited into the rehearsal space to help Club O' Noodles define Vietnamese American identity. I found this to be temporarily comforting, believing that Steve's presence as another non–Vietnamese American, Asian American person would somehow make my presence less conspicuous.

After an hour of my sitting, listening, and furiously writing down notes, a friendly voice rang out: "Oh, Yutian, we would really like to hear from you, too. Where are you in this picture? How do you envision your participation in the group?" I drew in a very deep breath, fidgeted in my chair, and straightened my back before attempting an answer. I tried to maintain the calm, collected, politically attuned graduate student/researcher/Asian American activist/dancer persona I had adopted in order to overcompensate for my ethnographic anxieties. Feeling embarrassed and feeling the need to say something "smart," I mumbled something about my desire to increase the visibility of Asian Americans in the arts by writing a history of Asian American performance that included Club O' Noodles.

As I mentioned earlier, I had been attending rehearsals for about a month and thought the best way for me to deal with the post-fieldwork writing of dispersing authority and representing multiple voices was to remain quiet. I was unsure how to negotiate a situation in which the members of the group were working to write a statement about how to portray themselves publicly. Would it be unfair for me to express how I thought they could most effectively market themselves, since the purpose of the workshop was to create a public image for people like myself to see? Was my proper role that of an insider or an outsider in this situation? What I did not anticipate was the fact that I was already integrated into the group. Unbeknownst to me, I was a member of Club O' Noodles. The conditions of my membership included my ambiguous identity as someone who kept bringing up the issue of being a researcher and not being completely part of the group. Yet, I had an excellent attendance record, seemed perfectly at ease in bare feet rolling around on the floor with everyone else, and seemed to enjoy doing mundane errands like carpooling, sweeping the rehearsal space floor, and collecting large stacks of newspapers.[4]

I misinterpreted the opportunity provided by Steve's workshop and believed I would actually hear the group's answer to "What is Vietnamese American identity?" or "How is Vietnamese American identity defined?" I do not mean to suggest that the group did not address the issue of Vietnamese American identity, but the workshop served the practical function of working out the mechanics of how the members would individually and collectively market something called "Vietnamese American performance." The workshop was comprised of two different discussions. The first discussion dealt with the issue of how individuals viewed their own participation in the group and the second discussion revolved around the identity of Club O' Noodles as an organization. The artistic director began the first discussion by asking how much time people were willing to commit to attending rehearsals, to performing, and to creating new material for future projects. Some people wanted to take on more administrative and leadership responsibilities, while others wanted to focus only on performing. One woman expressed interest in being part of the group on an intermittent basis so she could pursue other interests as well. She had originally joined for fun and did not anticipate how much time the rehearsal and performance schedule would require.

The issue of time commitment and degree of involvement became a central focus of this discussion. I could sense that some members were frustrated about the amount of time people were willing or able to commit to the organization. The director expressed feelings of abandonment by members who would leave after graduating from college to start "real" jobs. Most of the members in their early to mid-twenties were college students or recent college graduates, and others, in their mid- to late twenties, worked full time as teachers or social workers. I had to answer a direct question about how much time I was willing to spend attending rehearsals and whether or not I was going to learn roles and appear in performances. I told the group that I would attend workshops and rehearsals every weekend, but that I was not necessarily looking to be cast in productions.

My initial interest in attending rehearsals was to see *Laughter* again for the purpose of movement analysis and possibly to observe the choreographic process of any new Club O' Noodles work. In chapter 3, I described how, much to my surprise, CON spent a small percentage of their rehearsal time actually running through the performance itself. The same is true for their process of creating a new work. I had assumed that their creative process would somehow mirror my own past experiences, in which there was a correlation between improvisations and the actual material that found its way into a performance. I quickly discovered that this was not true for CON.

Since I was not planning to dance or act in any of the performances, I would choose moments to sit out and take notes during exercises or rehearsals that appeared more directly related to preparing for a specific performance. Sometimes it was difficult to differentiate between general process and performance-specific preparation, especially if material from the performance made its way into the check-in process. My participation level changed over time to include what Limón jokingly refers to as "less observation, more participation," or what Yvonne Daniel (1995) calls an "observing partici-pant."[5] By the end of 2000, I choreographed and performed in sections of the West Coast premiere of *Stories from a Nail Salon* (1999). This had to do with the fact that the group needed an extra body on stage, and not that the group's identity had become more ethnically expansive.

In the second half of the workshop, Steve taped a large piece of blank paper onto an easel and instructed everyone to say out loud words that they associated with Club O' Noodles. The words ranged from adjectives describing the political focus of the organization to specific activities that took place in rehearsal. The members used words that I loosely categorized under the following four categories: political, artistic, therapeutic, and recreational. The first words people offered fell under the "political" category. The company already employed terms like "bicultural," "empowerment," "activism," and "socially conscious" in their press releases and program notes, so it was not surprising to hear these words first.

Political	Artistic	Therapeutic	Recreational
Vietnamese	professional	peace of mind	retreat
immigrant	amateur	health	dreams
political force	collaborate	supportive	fun
American	expression	emotions	
activism	opportunity	understanding	
education	creativity	acknowledgement	
tolerance	rehearsal	unconditional	
biculturalism	artistic	together	
community	cultural	accepting	
empowerment	theater	constructive	
	experimenting	open	
	stories	inclusive	
	dance	therapy	
	music	sharing	
	workshops	passion	
	songs	friends	
		family	
		nurture	
		listening	
		being heard	
		affirmation	
		validation	
		sanctuary	

As people continued offering ideas, they fell increasingly in the categories I name "therapeutic." During rehearsal, people would often joke that Club O' Noodles was like a cult, poking fun at the ritual of checking in, in acknowledgment of its borderline association with group therapy. They called Club O' Noodles a "refuge" and even used the word "sanctuary." The words under the therapeutic category are suggestive of New Age therapy, yet the outward persona of the organization is unrelentingly political in terms of advocating an unromanticized vision of Vietnamese American cultural identity.

After the group finished the list, Steve wrote the word "refugee" next to "immigrant" and asked the group how the two words differed in meaning. Khan (a pseudonym) replied, "I used to think of myself as a refugee, but now I think of myself as an immigrant. [*pauses*] A refugee is someone who is at the mercy of the country that they are in." Someone else added, " 'Refugee' connotes desperation." Khan equated the word immigrant with belonging: "An immigrant is someone with legal status and is allowed to be in the United States, unlike a refugee who has no choice in the matter." Steve pointed out to the group that the refugee experience differentiates Vietnamese Americans from other Asian Americans in the United States.[6] In prompting Club O' Noodles's members to define their difference from other Asian Americans, Steve asked the group to destabilize unified notions of pan–Asian American identity, even though the collective never used the term "Asian American" to describe themselves. Steve made a point to emphasize the fact that defining the organization as "Vietnamese American" is what makes Club O' Noodles special. Unsaid but implied in Steve's remark was that in order for Club O' Noodles to claim a Vietnamese American identity, it would also need to embrace a refugee identity.

The discussion continued among the members around the definitions of refugee and immigrant, and each individual's relationships to the terms. About two-thirds of the members considered themselves refugees, having lived in refugee camps as teenagers and children, while others considered themselves immigrants. Steve turned the discussion toward "The Boat Dance" in *Laughter,* stating that it was an important part of the show. Several of the members quickly agreed and described this particular section of the performance as the heart and soul of *Laughter*. They expressed a feeling of psychic and kinetic connection to the movements and the sound. One of the members who had been quiet during the discussion up until that moment began to look a bit uncomfortable as he said, "My relationship to 'The Boat Dance'? I'm not a boat person. I guess I'm lucky. I came to America on a plane after all of that." There was a moment of uncomfortable silence, as if no one knew how to integrate this disclosure into the greater claim that refugees and boat people distinguish Vietnamese Americans from other Asian Americans.

I looked around the room as everyone sat in silence, and my mind worked in overdrive. In my notes I wrote, "Okay, this is when someone is supposed acknowledge that while many are, not all Vietnamese people in the U.S. came as refugees; or that it's obvious that the subject requires more discussion; or ask what the trope of the refugee represents and what does it mean to reclaim or distance oneself from it." Always conscious of the amount of time different individuals talked during discussions, I refrained from jumping in to fill the silence. The silence suggested that although the company found the refugee experience an important theme to address in their work, it was not an all-encompassing identity for the entire group, but functioned as something that tied individuals to one another in different ways. There were the two members who one day discovered "Oh my God, we were on the same boat!"—while another two had found themselves responsible at age fourteen for filling out all the paperwork necessary to sponsor the rest of their families in Vietnam to join them in the United States. As the time allotted for the workshop was nearing its end, the discussion came to a close without any specific resolution.

If, during the discussion, the members were careful to name the differences in the group, in practice, Club O' Noodles continued to rehearse *Laughter* under the assumption that everyone had the right to embody particular stories on stage. During one of the rehearsals that took place after the workshop with Steve, I was asked to work with one group of performers to help clean up the choreography for "The Boat Dance" in preparation for a performance in San Jose, California. In addition, one of the key female members would not be able to perform, so I was asked to take on some of her minor roles. Although the group stuck to the practice of giving everyone an opportunity to lead the group during check-in and warm-ups, the director assigned people specific roles when it came time to rehearse scenes or songs in a performance.

Since I had attended several performances of *Laughter,* I knew the script and choreography fairly well; the director would have me watch run-throughs of the performance to give the cast feedback on timing and spacing. Over time, I worked as the rehearsal director for anything that involved movement, including "The Boat Dance." I was nervous about directing and performing in this particular section of the show, especially after the members themselves expressed having such a personal connection to the material. To add to my anxiety, "The Boat Dance" occurred in the middle of *Laughter,* sandwiched between two scenes that posed ideological critiques of representational systems. As I discussed in chapter 2, the choreography of "The Boat Dance" in *Laughter* evoked physical memories of thirst, hunger, and psychic displacement—a literal drifting in the middle of nowhere.

I found myself faced with the task not only of having to perform but also of redirecting what were clearly someone else's bodily memories. I finally asked the dancers in my group how they generated the original movement vocabulary for "The Boat Dance." The movement originated from a series of workshops led by Nobuko Miyamoto, a pioneer of Asian American performance.[7] Those who had worked on the original performance described the workshops as intensely emotional and recounted how Miyamoto asked those who did escape Vietnam by boat to physicalize what it was like to sit on a boat with no food, water, or knowledge of where they would end up. These memories translated into movement motifs that were then integrated into an improvisational structure.

The choreographic structure was simple. The dancers were divided into two groups of four. Within each group, the dancers were arranged in a diamond formation and each dancer had to follow the movement of whoever was in front of the group. If the leader made a 180-degree turn, then the person who was originally in the back of the diamond formation would become the new leader. Basically, if there was no one in front of you, you were the leader. From the audience's perspective, the group looked as if it were performing a predetermined sequence of movements in unison. In actuality, the piece was composed as a structured improvisation. Since I was the newest person to learn the movement vocabulary, I was placed at the front of the diamond formation facing the audience so that I would not have to worry about following the movement at the beginning of the dance. This meant I had to establish the tempo and the mood of the group's movement.

During dress rehearsal on stage, someone yelled out, "Remember what it was like to be on the boat!" Maybe it was my lack of imagination, but I found myself unable or perhaps unwilling to call forth such an emotional state. Instead, I used my three rehearsals to learn the movement vocabulary of the other performers by imitating their form, shape, energy, and speed, and found myself questioning the politics of inter-ethnic casting in a situation where my body was not visually differentiated from the rest of the cast. After the show, a middle-aged couple approached me to tell me how wonderful the performance had been. They were especially moved at how accurately we portrayed the experience of the boat people and how meaningful it was to see Vietnamese people on stage. It was one of those post-show moments when one wants to bask in the glory of post-show compliments, yet I was compelled to disappoint—to disclose the fact that I am not Vietnamese American.

People's desire to see authentic Vietnamese American bodies performing

Vietnamese American experiences was an important recruitment tool for Club O' Noodles. During a conversation I had with Lily (a pseudonym), she reflected on seeing *Laughter* for the first time, believing it to be an accurate portrayal of her own personal experiences. She felt that only other Vietnamese Americans could have represented the stories she saw. In particular, she was surprised at the accuracy of the sewing scenes, in which the mother enlists the help of all the children. Lily explained that she spent much of her childhood feeling ashamed of her family, believing that they were the only people in America who sewed clothing for a living. Whenever her family looked for a house to rent, the house had to have an attached garage so that the family could park inside the garage and unload all the bags of fabric without the neighbors seeing.

Lily admitted that before she joined Club O' Noodles she was so ashamed of what her family did for a living that she never told anyone until one of her friends came to see her perform. After the show, her friend approached her and said, "How did you know my family did that?" This moment of recognition redolent with the desire for authenticity reflects an earlier moment in Asian American studies, in which the "true" story of the Asian American experience could emerge. Contemporary Asian American cultural studies claims, with its critique of cultural nationalism, to move away from authenticity. In its place, a method of reading Asian American cultural production as that which troubles and resists notions of unified or essentialized Asian American identities has emerged.

The desire for authenticity, in the spirit of Frank Chin and James Moy, has come to signify dated approaches to Asian American cultural production. Lily's reactions to Club O' Noodles's work demonstrates the continued relevance of the authentic. Despite theoretical moves to read Asian American cultural production outside of critiques of authenticity, in practice a strong desire still remains to see and designate authentic representations and authentic bodies.

In Jude Narita's one-woman show, *Coming into Passion/Song for a Sansei* (1987), she portrays a wide range of characters, including a nervous, middle-aged nisei woman; a rebellious, teenage sansei girl; a blind Cambodian woman; and a fast-talking Vietnamese prostitute. A pioneer in Asian American solo performance, Narita was one of the early performance artists who brought the complexity of Asian American women's lives onto the stage. The work was extremely successful on the college touring circuit where I first saw her work (at the University of California–Davis, in 1991). I remember the performance quite vividly, especially the throng of inspired Asian American female students (including myself) who rushed up to the stage. Narita had staged and put into practice in a very public way the ideas that we had encountered in a fledgling Asian American studies program on campus. In the early 1990s, her performance workshop for Asian American women at the University of California–Los Angeles was instrumental in launching the careers of a second generation of performance artists, including Denise Uyehara.

A decade later, Narita would become part of the establishment in the Asian American performance art scene, and the reputation of her work would shift. One Saturday afternoon while Lily and I were driving home after another rehearsal, the subject of Narita's newest show, *Walk the Mountain,* came up.[8] Based on Narita's research in Vietnam and Cambodia, *Walk the Mountain* deals with Vietnamese and Cambodian women's wartime memories and postwar experiences. The most notable character includes a doctor who cares for children born with severe birth defects caused by Agent Orange and other war-related environmental contaminants.

I asked Lily if she was planning to see *Walk the Mountain*. She said, "No, I'm not going to see a show by that woman." I asked her what she meant by "that woman." Lily replied that she found Narita's portrayal of a Vietnamese prostitute in *Coming into Passion* "annoying." She emphasized the fact that Vietnamese women have been so closely associated with prostitution that Narita's portrayal was a cliché. Moreover, Lily felt betrayed that Narita, as an Asian woman, did not only play the role, but had, in fact, authored the role.

Lily viewed Narita's ability to envision multiple and nuanced experiences of Japanese American women across multiple generations in stark contrast with her choice to depict a prostitute as the singular representation of Vietnamese women. Portrayed without a clearly defined relationship to the United States, the prostitute appears out of place within a narrative arc that situates the rest of the characters as citizens, immigrants, or refugees. Uncontextualized but unmistakably foreign, Narita's prostitute longs for her American "boyfriend," who gives her presents. For Lily, the idea of having to watch Narita perform an entire evening of work about Vietnamese women felt tiresome given the similarities between Narita's portrayal of the Vietnamese prostitute and that of *Miss Saigon*.

Lily was not the first to have a problem with Narita's character of the prostitute. During the post-show discussion in 1991 at UC Davis, a woman brought up that very issue and asked Narita if she thought she was reinforcing stereotypes of Asian women by choosing to include the character of a Vietnamese prostitute. Narita seemed prepared for the question and stated that it was something that many people ask her during the post-show discussion. She emphasized her desire to give the women who work as prostitutes a voice. She believed it was important to acknowledge the fact that there are Vietnamese women who do work as prostitutes. Her goal in portraying the character was to make visible a woman with aspirations and vulnerabilities who happens to be a sex worker and not to embody a representation of sex work itself. In other words, despite audiences' discomfort with and objections to the character over the years, Narita continued to keep the character in the performance.

In the late '90s and at the turn of the millennium, Club O' Noodles and Narita were part of the same Asian American performance scene in Los Angeles; they performed in the same venues and in the same performance series, like Highways Performance Space's "Treasure in the House," and also competed for overlapping Asian American audiences. Lily's objection to Narita's portrayal of a Vietnamese prostitute speaks to the issue of authenticity in terms of the politics of representation and the politics of who does the representing. Lily's impatience with the trope of the prostitute itself is understandable, given the long-standing tradition of using prostitutes to stand in for Asian women in film, television, and the stage.

From a pan–Asian Americanist point of view, Narita's attempt to disentangle the trope of normative Asian female sexuality from prostitution without ascribing asexuality is theoretically noteworthy; however, from Lily's point of view as a Vietnamese American woman, the move was unpalatable and unproductive. Narita's effort to empower the Vietnamese prostitute did not manifest itself as empowerment for the Vietnamese American women watching the production. Lily and her friends did not identify with nor empathize with the representation that Narita offered. The prostitute in Narita's performance remains a singular point of contention and makes visible the limits of the pan–Asian Americanist ethos in her work.

These two examples—Steve's workshop and the reactions to Narita's performances—mark out the contours of belonging and the work of self-representation. They underscore the labors of producing an institution defined as "Vietnamese American" and the naturalized assumptions of belonging. Given that Club O' Noodles's work is based on questions of belonging, the idea of belonging can be extended to the role of a researcher. What counts as "presence"? Performers like to think of presence as performance quality that separates the good from the mediocre. Since it is often spoken of in metaphysical terms—that which cannot be taught—how should one account for one's presence as a researcher when called forth to perform? The desire to blend into the walls—in other words, to disavow one's bodily presence—and witness events at hand conflicts with the expectation to be fully present when called upon to participate and take one's turn to perform.

Working on Class

If the public portrayal of Vietnamese experiences of the U.S. war in Vietnam and of the harrowing experiences of the boat people served as a communal focal point for collective healing, then rehearsals for *Stories from a Nail Salon* tested the limits of cohesion. *Stories from a Nail Salon* examines the psychic costs of Vietnamese American involvement in the nail salon industry. According to *Nails* (a trade publication for the nail care industry), an estimated 40 percent of U.S. manicurists are of Vietnamese descent and 80 percent of nail salons are Vietnamese American–owned businesses.[9] The Vietnamese American presence in the nail salon industry has spawned its own publication, *Viet Salon*. In her 2007 article "Inside the Vietnamese Salon," reporter Tara Bui recounts an American success story in which two brothers, Robert and Vu Nguyen, surmount obstacles, including gender discrimination, to become award-winning nail artists whose high-end manicures command top dollar in the industry.[10] If the Nguyen brothers' story, a tale of both economic success and professional fulfillment, makes nail salon work a socially acceptable profession within Vietnamese American communities, Club O' Noodles's research uncovered a different story.

The structure of the performance of *Nail Salon* was conceived by filmmaker Ham Tran, and inspired by Hung Nguyen's desire to confront his own class-based shame in regard to nail salon work. Nguyen admitted that even though he understood why members of his family worked as nail technicians, he nevertheless felt ashamed of them. Other members of Club O'

Noodles expressed similar feelings. Although nail salon work represented a step up from piecework (sewing), Nguyen characterized working in a nail salon as Vietnamese immigrants' last-ditch effort to "make it" in America when all else has failed. The work promised the dream of financial success, but for the most part it represented monotonous and toxic work. Although hip to the oppressive forces of self-internalized model-minority discourse, Nguyen identified class identity as the underlying source of his embarrassment. Even if working in and then owning a nail salon could prove lucrative, it is not considered a proper middle-class occupation—a sentiment echoed by Lily, a graduate of an elite private college, who hid her family's work history from her friends.

More than any other time, the workshops that the group conducted for *Nail Salon* prior to working on the show itself revealed the extent to which class identity would prove to be an issue that divided the company. As an organization of artists working on the margins of dancetheater and the Vietnamese American community, Club O' Noodles consistently struggled to resist the pressure of succumbing to self-internalized "proper" model-minority behavior. Model-minority stereotypes proved difficult to avoid as class-based prejudices emerged through discourses of shame. The *Nail Salon* project differed from *Laughter* because the themes and experiences portrayed in *Laughter* were drawn from the performers' own life experiences. Material for *Stories from a Nail Salon* came from interviews with nail salon workers, including former Club O' Noodles's members who had gone to work in the nail salon industry.

Hung Nguyen and Ham Tram went so far as to learn how to "do nails" by working in a nail salon. The initial conversations about the piece brought into focus class conflicts among workers in a nail salon and between owners of nail salons and their workers. Several performers related stories in which workers' responses to underemployment were often the cause of class conflicts. For example, Lily's mother Lan (a pseudonym) worked as a schoolteacher in Vietnam before coming to the United States. Lan, who was well educated and spoke English, was surprised to find that in the United States she could not even find a job as a teacher's aide, and resorted to "doing nails" in order to support the family. Lan resented taking orders from younger female co-workers whom she thought were less educated or came from lower-class families, and felt that the job was beneath her.

Nguyen and Tran were also interested in the racism within the nail salon industry, in which "legitimate" white manicurists felt anger and resentment toward the competition posed by increasing numbers of Vietnamese American–owned nail salons. Accusations of unsanitary conditions, coupled with reports that Vietnamese nail salons drive down the prices of manicures and pedicures, echoed the charges motivating late-nineteenth- and twentieth-century anti-Asian labor laws. Rather than dwelling on mainstream stereotypes projected onto the Vietnamese nail salon, the performers directed their resentment at the exploitive nature of the work environment regulated by Vietnamese American business owners who employ their fellow ethnics in less-than-ideal working conditions.

Clearly frustrated by a system in which an individual has little choice but to work in a nail salon, some of the performers complained about the willingness of Vietnamese workers to remain in soul-deadening and toxic work conditions. The company members themselves were conflicted over doing nails. Some identified nail salon work as simply quick, tax-free money, while others blamed the obsession over money for causing the destruction of Vietnamese American families. One person blamed increasing rates of Vietnamese American juvenile delinquency on parents whose efforts to become model minorities mistake economic success for parental guidance. Another reported an incident in which she discovered her neighbor's child with his head stuck between the bars of a wrought-iron door. She was angry at the parents for leaving the child unattended and angry that the parents were trapped in a system in which their livelihood depended on working long hours. In these emotionally charged discussions, the boundaries between exploitative working conditions, institutionalized racism, speculations, and anecdotal evidence were blurred and these factors were oftentimes conflated with one another. It was clear from the discussions that the performance piece was going to force Vietnamese American audiences to face some very unpopular and pointed questions about the human costs of the Vietnamese nail salon industry.

In many ways, Club O' Noodles's treatment of labor in *Laughter* dealt with the issue of appearance. The failure to secure model-minority occupations sparked intergenerational conflicts between immigrant parents and their children. In *Laughter,* when a son refuses to help his mother sew and declares that he is going to work in a nail salon, his father rages. Club O'

Noodles's references to low-paid labor such as sewing provide a counter-representation to universalized narratives of Asian American success. In *Laughter,* sewing is not portrayed as a dead-end job or a last resort. However embarrassing, it is framed as a secret beginning done in the privacy of one's home. Sewing is renarrativized as a noble endeavor, once subject to *Laughter*'s critique of capital, in which immigrant women and children, who sew the clothes, receive $1.50 per item for wares that are sold in department stores for $50. In contrast, working in a nail salon makes visible one's disappointments, failures, and unfulfilled ambitions.

The exploitative nature of piecework is quantifiable in terms of the cost-to-profit ratio, as is the unmistakable reference to critiques of multinational companies who use child labor to produce cheap goods for the U.S. market. Nail salons are associated with skilled labor (one needs to be licensed), beauty, and fashion; and though this service-oriented work takes place in sweatshop-like working conditions, such conditions are masked by the shopping malls and middle-class neighborhoods in which salons are often located. On the surface, the laboring bodies do not appear exploited; yet, owning a nail salon does not quite fit the requirements of inclusion in the ranks of "real" model-minority professionalism.

Workshopping Class

The process of creating *Nail Salon* provided a more complex picture than *Laughter* of how the group perceived the relationship between class and the body. Nguyen invited Mark (a pseudonym), a well-known, Los Angeles–based Asian American performance artist, to teach a series of workshops to help the company generate material for the nail salon project. It was common practice for Club O' Noodles to draw upon the larger network of Asian American performance artists to present workshops, so that the group could learn techniques that it could readily incorporate into the rehearsal process. Artists were chosen for their ability to present material that could help Club O' Noodles in some way to improve the working process of the group, develop a performance skill, or generate material useful to a performance.

Mark's workshop centered on discussing issues of difference and the effect of class identity. Rather than discussing difference in depersonalized, theoretical terms, Mark asked the performers to discuss their own sense of class identity, how this had affected their perception of their own ethnic identity, and how this in turn affected their perceptions of other people. Instead of championing romantic notions of difference as a celebratory theoretical given, this exercise revealed the ways in which unspoken class prejudices between members of the group were oftentimes masked as differences in personality. The process also exposed how class identity was intertwined with the perceived success of assimilation into American culture, and particularly how the stereotype of the "whitewashed" Vietnamese American citizen is pitted against the fresh-off-the-boat immigrant.

We were asked to write the following information on a piece of paper: our full name, ethnic background, class identity, a family object that represented our class background, and some important individual characteristic about ourselves that we believed went unnoticed or were downplayed by other people. We spent about fifteen minutes writing. Mark then asked each of us, one at a time, to introduce ourselves to the group based on the information we had written. The rest of the group was instructed to listen to the speaker and write down anything that sounded interesting for future use as material in a performance.

The exercise was designed so that people could hear how others interpreted the categories, since everyone's interpretation of what constitutes "ethnic" and "class identity" varied. The exercise displayed a diverse set of conditions for defining "Vietnamese American." Differences in ethnic identification, language ability, class, religion, and how each individual came to the United States destabilized the term "Vietnamese American" as a unifying identity, since each individual created the conditions for his or her own definition. Each member's disidentification worked to take apart Club O' Noodles's carefully crafted and unified identity as Vietnamese American, which Club O' Noodles used to differentiate itself from other Asian American performance groups. Since multicultural programming operates on the practice of filling niches, calling attention to the group's Vietnamese American–ness is both artistically and politically strategic for writing grant proposals and marketing performances.

People's explanations for their ethnic identities centered on genealogy. Most members considered themselves Vietnamese, though some would report having a distant relative who was ethnically Chinese. Another reported a rumored French ancestor. Eric (a pseudonym) revealed that his ethnic identity changed depending on where his family lived: "My family was originally from China, but in Vietnam, we were Vietnamese. We spoke Vietnamese, ate Vietnamese food, and were Vietnamese. But all of a sudden when we came to America, we became Chinese." Someone asked him how this affected the way in which he related to Club O' Noodles as a Vietnamese American performance group. Eric's cultural affinity with the group centered on remembering that he, too, had learned the Vietnamese lullabies sung in *Laughter,* and several of the characters portrayed in the performance reminded him of his own family.

Eric's sense of ethnic ambiguity questions the parameters of what constitutes "cultural identity." Eric's ability to suddenly become culturally Chinese after growing up in and identifying with Vietnam suggests that ethnic identity is strongly tied to biological origins. Or is it that U.S. racial discourse regarding racialized ethnic identity forces simplistic notions of cultural identity? Eric's Chinese Vietnamese identity is unreadable within a racial/ethnic infrastructure that still reduces multicultural identity to biological difference. His multicultural body does not provide biological proof of multiple identities in the absence of a history of interracial and interethnic sex as genetic evidence. Discourses of transnationalism do not necessarily solve this problem. Transnationalism implies constant travel back and forth between places. For Eric, his Chinese-ness emerged as a result of spatial and temporal distance from Vietnam.

Allen Chun (1996) questions the entire concept of Chinese ethnic identity and locates the fallacy of using "Chinese-ness" as an ethnic identity by calling attention to the situation in China, where there is no notion of Chinese-ness as an ethnic identity. Instead, Chinese-ness is a modern idea that describes a national identity tied to political ideology. In Taiwan, Chinese identity is tied to a past cultural history and also to a political ideology that is still legally at war with the ideology of the People's Republic of China. He goes through the list of permutations of how Chinese-ness is used to demarcate an ethnic identity that does not necessarily exist in the geographical center from where it is supposed to derive (111–38).

Chun's dismantling of Chinese-ness identifies structures invested in the maintenance of the national identity as a conflated ethnic identity in the diaspora. Lisa Lowe (1996) argues that Asian immigrant populations in America do not necessarily choose to retain ethnic and racial identity out of a desire to maintain cultural heritage, and that the practice is a legacy of U.S.

legislation: laws barring Asian immigrants from citizenship, Asian immigrant exclusion acts, and national origins quotas. Despite changes in naturalization and immigration laws in the latter half of the twentieth century, Asian Americans are still haunted by this history and are not fully incorporated into a national American cultural and political identity. Left out of late-nineteenth-century and early-twentieth-century melting pot and cultural pluralist rhetoric that sought to domesticate the influx of European immigrants, Asian Americans are forced to contend with their "perpetual foreignness." The success of European immigration immortalized by Ellis Island functions as the symbolic cornerstone in demonstrating the effectiveness of democratic U.S. ideals and the nation's ability to "overlook" ethnic difference and willingness not to consider it a social impediment. For Asian Americans, ethnicity functions as code for racial difference and becomes a conceptual category useful for identifying reasons for exclusion.

For Club O' Noodles to articulate intra-ethnic differences that reveal prejudicial attitudes risks destroying its own project of advocating for Vietnamese American subjectivity. To admit that Asian Americans harbor racism toward each other "proves" that Asian Americans are just as racist, classist, or sexist as unenlightened white individuals and therefore do not deserve recognition as an oppressed racial minority. This equalizing logic threatens the gravity of even the most obvious evidence of anti-Asian violence and imagery. At the same time, the denial of intra- and inter-ethnic differences allows for social injustices to continue within communities. Issues of domestic violence, child abuse, homophobia, and economic exploitation go unnoticed in an attempt to maintain a politically unified community.

During Mark's workshop, the group established that ethnic identity alone could not account for the multitude of life experiences, and class identity took on a more central role in conversations regarding how people viewed themselves within a Vietnamese American social context. In this session, the group moved away from a unified understanding of Vietnamese American-ness provided by a racialized ethnic identity, in order to discuss the implications of unspoken conflicts created by class difference. Stripped of its status as a marker of specialness, ethnicity gave way to class as a potentially divisive topic of discussion.

The discussion of class identity continued at the next meeting. Mark played an assortment of sounds and music; he asked people to embody their own class identity in response and to dance as a character with that identity. Confused, people had a difficult time coming up with a physicalization of class identity. Several people resorted to pantomiming activities associated with the music. For example, when Mark played classical music, some people mimed the act of sitting and listening to music with a look of enjoyment while others mimicked boredom and distaste. Mark then drew an imaginary line down the center of the room and designated one end of the line "lower class" and the other end, "upper class." He instructed everyone to stand on the line according to how one saw oneself on the class continuum. Everyone milled around for a few minutes, then finally grouped themselves into three clusters on the line. Mark asked us to look around and see where we had all placed ourselves, and talk to the people nearest to us about why they had placed themselves in those spots.

Having to embody one's class identity generated tension within the group, something that did not occur the day before. In the previous meeting, people related stories of how their class identities changed depending on their family's wartime financial situation. For some of the performers, their own current financial standing defined their class identity, while others associated their class with their childhood upbringing. People also equated class with education, either with their own level or with a familial history of accumulated educational achievements. Identifying class with financial success made class identity a transient state. A few members related stories of drastic changes in their families' social status before and after the war in Vietnam, as well as before and after they arrived in the United States.

Most of those stories did not necessarily follow the model-minority "rags to riches" narrative; but rather, in fact, undermined it. As a whole, the stories revealed that, in many cases, attempts to articulate class identity produced expressions of sentiment—as in feelings of entitlement, or feelings of having to overcome insurmountable obstacles. Lily, a schoolteacher, considered her current situation as solidly middle class and resented the fact that her mother instilled upper-class values in the family despite their working-class economic situation. She cited the contradiction between class identity and reality as the reason why, as a child, she was embarrassed by her family members' occupations.

As the day wore on, the discussion of how one's family (which people interpreted as one's parents) perceived class identity turned toward individuals' perceptions of her or his own class identity. This is when people became noticeably uncomfortable and tension began building within the group, making it increasingly difficult to discuss class. The exercise forced the group to confront class prejudices in a social context that on the previous day had appeared uniformly middle class. It revealed the limits of political consciousness within Club O' Noodles when it came to class identity. The group's performance activities represented a clear antiracist imagery, but the issue of class differences could not be addressed within a coalition based solely on ethnic affinities. Having three clusters of people identify themselves as working-class, middle-class, and upper-class subjects forced the group to create visible categories of "us" and "them."

Carl (a pseudonym) walked to his end of the line, designated as "upper class," and I stood next to him. I was a graduate student and the only person in the room whose job it was to spend all my waking hours "studying performance." While others spoke of juggling work, school, and rehearsal, I juggled teaching dance, reading and writing about dance, and attending rehearsals as my work. Carl was the only other person in the room who did not have a "day job," and managed to support himself as a full-time artist through a combination of grants, teaching, and performing.

After we divided ourselves into three groups, Mark directed us to discuss within our groups why we decided to stand where we did. Carl and I faced each other to talk; it soon became apparent from our discussion that we both assumed a sense of entitlement to "art." Our involvement in making art was not entirely from an altruistic sense of community, as outlined in Club O' Noodles's mission statement; rather, in the back of our minds, we still had a desire for the modernist notion of the "art object"—in this case, self-consciously experimental performance as an end unto itself. Our sense of class privilege provided the leap of faith needed to pursue a career in experimental performance. As we talked, it became increasingly evident that we had also knowingly chosen a career path with unpredictable financial reward, thus failing to guarantee our inherited class identity (in the economic sense).

The other two groups were much larger and we could sense everyone looking around to see where people decided to stand. What stood out was the fact that the majority of the members identified themselves as belonging to the middle class, even though most criticized middle-class identity as some sort of undeserved privilege. Within the context of social justice, the material indicators of middle-class values (driving cars and living in suburban housing developments) symbolized anonymous and impersonal forces of oppression. It soon became clear that the critique of class called forth an imagined middle-class Asian American subject demonized for its perceived passivity, undeserved privilege, and proximity to the model-minority stereotype. Given the ubiquity of the model-minority stereotype, there was an unspoken anxiety that evidence of an Asian American middle class could invalidate hard-won claims to institutional racism. Ironically, it was this middle-class privilege that allowed the group access to resources needed to negotiate for rehearsal space, secure contracts for performances, and network with a larger middle-class performance community.

Upon closer examination, most people also defined class privilege through educational and not financial status. Almost all of the members had or were working toward college degrees. However, there were wide discrepancies between where one went to school (a public teaching institution in the California state university system; a research institution in the University of California system; or a private liberal arts college), how one paid for it (student loans, part-time or full-time jobs), and how included one felt within various levels of the campus community.

To expose class privilege is both necessary and risky for communities of color, particularly for Asian Americans. It is risky because in the face of anti-Asian sentiment, the model-minority stereotype has consistently provided an argument for an Asian American presence in the United States based on perceived economic productivity. The media heralds Vietnamese immigrants as the ultimate model minority. Since the Vietnam War functions as an icon for U.S. guilt, the success of Vietnamese immigrants is economic proof of U.S. altruism and works as a bargaining chip for forgiveness. The discussion of class is necessary because the homogenization of normative middle-class Asian America implies that Asians are absent from the full range of American cultural and political life because of inherent cultural differences. In other words, with the assumption that Asian Americans possess uniformly distributed economic resources, feelings of alienation cannot be explained by economic deprivation. Alienation must then result from unalterable cultural differences, based on either a genetic predilection to resist adaptation or an overdetermined sense of group identity that disables an individual's ability to wholly embrace the process of becoming an "independent American."

After everyone made known their class identities, Mark asked for two volunteers from different class backgrounds to pair up and talk to one another about the positive and negatives aspects of their class identities. He instructed the rest of us to listen and take notes. Tuyen (middle class) and Vuong (working class) volunteered (both are pseudonyms). Tuyen made the following comments: "Middle-class people don't want problems of the poor. The unknown is scary. Middle-class people like comfort and stability. Middle-class people want to help through churches and non-profits." In response, Vuong commented on Tuyen's remarks, "It hurts to hear that poor people are problems and that all poor people are in gangs or homeless. Wealthy people also rob and do drugs." Obviously, Vuong felt labeled by Tuyen's comments. Mark attempted to redirect the conversation and asked Vuong to talk about himself and not respond to what Tuyen said. The conversation continued for another ten minutes, until Vuong accused Tuyen of labeling working-class people, and Tuyen said that he felt guilty about his middle-class privilege. Finally, Carl blew up and demanded that the conversation stop. Mark called for an end to the exercise; the group decided that it was time to end the meeting.

During the check-out, Carl explained that he felt angry that the conversation had deteriorated into blame and self-pity. He felt that the conversation was going nowhere and that both people were set up to encourage and reiterate class stereotypes. Carl perceived the exercise as a failure because both parties blamed their own class identity as grounds for feeling oppressed. Vuong said he had sensed that he needed to fight against Tuyen. The group did not discuss the fact that each person used differing criteria to define his or her own class identity. Vuong and Tuyen ended up talking about class in nonspecific terms, trapped in a series of clichés. As a result, Tuyen succumbed to guilt and Vuong, feeling labeled, became defensive. One could also interpret the session as a success in terms of making class prejudice visible, but Carl believed that the two had no choice but to reproduce the stereotypes. To complicate the situation further, it was Carl, self-identified as upper class, and not the other participants, who ultimately called for an end to the discussion. I felt I had finally witnessed the limits of Club O' Noodles-as-therapy. With class lines in high relief, this session tested the farthest reaches of confession and disclosure as productive and affirming practices. Sharing is not always an easy or positive experience.

Contrary to what one might expect after a contentious rehearsal, the lines of communication in Club O' Noodles did not break down; the group continued to convene and work on *Nail Salon*. The ritual check-out offered people an opportunity to comment on the events of the day. In a telling fashion, someone finally commented on my note taking. Carl told the group that as he was becoming increasingly annoyed by Vuong and Tuyen's argument, there was a moment when "I looked over at Yutian and all I could think was 'What is that damn woman scribbling in her notebook? I mean, what could she be possibly writing down at a time like this?'"

Carl's question has to do with what is worth representing. What I have attempted to represent in this chapter, through an ethnographic reading of Club O' Noodles's rehearsal process, is an extension of José Muñoz's metaphorical use of disidentification to demonstrate the actual struggle for self-representation, which includes false starts. I have also attempted to leave traces of my own body in this account, to make evident the researcher's impact on the subject of study. Even as I attempted to simply observe the action unfolding between Vuong and Tuyen, just as everyone else was doing, my presence was called out. It was not because I looked asleep, got up to go the bathroom, answered my pager, or opened a bag of chips, as some of the others present did. It was my writing body that gave me away. I was sitting upright, legs crossed, notebook in lap, paying close attention, and scribbling away. In this moment, even after all of this inclusion, my body gave me away as I performed the role of the researcher and failed to pass as a member of Club O' Noodles.

5

WRITING *NAIL SALON*

The following analysis of *Stories from a Nail Salon* differs from my reading of *Laughter* in that it takes into account my presence during the early stages of the development of its West Coast premiere at Highways Performance Space in November 1999. When I started working with Club O' Noodles in 1996, the company had already set about making plans to create a piece about the social and economic phenomenon of Vietnamese American–owned nail salons. Written by Ham Tran and codirected by Hung Nguyen and Hiep Nguyen, *Stories from a Nail Salon* was first produced at the New World Theater in Amherst, Massachusetts, as part of a Vietnamese American performance series. After the initial production, the group returned to California to revise the production and prepare for its West Coast premiere.

By 1999, I had appeared in one performance of *Laughter,* taking on small, nonspeaking roles and filling in as an extra for scenes requiring several bodies on stage. In the months leading up to *Nail Salon*'s premiere, Nguyen asked me if I was planning on performing in the new version of the show. I agreed to assist as a rehearsal director in charge of all the choreographed movement sections of the show.[1] For the East Coast version, Maura Nguyen Donohue, the director of the New York City–based In Mixed Company, choreographed several sections of *Nail Salon.* The California cast differed from the East Coast cast, so many of the members could not remember the specifics of the choreography. Since not much rehearsal time remained to work with all of the new cast simultaneously, I decided to compartmentalize the choreography.

Instead of trying to reconstruct the timing and phrasing of movements from videotaped footage of the East Coast show, then reteaching them to everyone, I asked the members to show me anything they could remember, particularly the motifs that they felt were visually central to the movement sequences. Club O' Noodles planned to undertake a major revision of *Nail Salon* for the West Coast premiere, but I wanted to find a way to maintain the performers' emotional connection to the movements generated from their residency at the New World Theater. After learning the phrases and motifs that they remembered, I restructured the choreography to fit the needs of the piece (time, space, number of dancers).

One challenge of working with the new cast was distance. One of the newest cast members lived in northern California, so I would not have an opportunity to work with her until the night of the dress rehearsal. In order to accommodate people's schedules, I took a cue from the Club O' Noodles's working process and built an improvisatory element into the choreography. Club O' Noodles had been using this choreographic structure quite successfully in *Laughter* in anticipation of an ever-changing cast. As a group, Club O' Noodles worked under the assumption that everyone could execute any part of the performance, regardless of technical ability. With the approach of the opening and the need to account for variation in the performers' skill levels, I faced the challenge of crafting a movement vocabulary that everyone could master in a fairly short amount of time.

From past experience working with the group, I knew the choreography had to accommodate last-minute changes in the cast with relative ease. The cast member living in northern California was a highly accomplished actor, but her having to absorb choreography without the opportunity to rehearse proved a challenge. It was unthinkable for anyone to suggest that she not appear in any of the scenes; so the aesthetic choices I made were designed to accommodate Club O' Noodles's ethos of inclusion in its definition of "community theater."

In addition to choreographing the movement sequences, I continued to observe rehearsals of other scenes. Instead of taking my usual field notes, I fed lines and wrote notes for the performers, with suggestions and corrections on spacing, timing, and overall performance quality. As opening night loomed, Club O' Noodles increased its rehearsals from one or two a week to four or five. The increase included rehearsals for individuals to work on specific sections of the performance. At this time, I was only able to commit to one additional evening rehearsal in addition to the normal weekend rehearsal. So, for the first time, the director scheduled some rehearsals around what the company needed me to accomplish. Because of this, there were some parts of the performance that I was intimately familiar with and others I never saw rehearsed. This process differed from my experience of watching *Laughter,* which I was able to see rehearsed in its entirety.

Unable to attend the opening weekend of *Stories from a Nail Salon*, I planned to see the show during the second of its two-weekend run at Highways. A few days before the second weekend of the show, I received a frantic phone call from Ham Tran, the playwright. One of the female performers had a scheduling conflict and could no longer perform for the duration of the run. There was, however, some good news. Prior to the opening, the director found a new cast member, Jane (pseudonym), to play the part of The Popular Culture Queen. Jane was also willing to take on the much larger role of Thuy. And here was the catch: for her to play Thuy, the director needed someone else to perform the role of The Popular Culture Queen, who makes several brief appearances, including a jazzy, Las Vegas show–style routine. As part of my rehearsal duties, I had reconstructed this routine for Club O' Noodles. Tran called me first, assuming that I would not have to learn the choreography since I had taught it to the group.

After agreeing to perform in the show, due to open in two days, I hung up the phone and began panicking. Choreographing and performing are two different skills. Ham was right, I knew the material; however, the movement was created on the bodies of the performers present during rehearsal, which meant I had tailored the vocabulary, phrasing, and attack to make each dancer look as good as possible given the varying technical proficiencies of group members. After I set the phrasing, timing, and spacing of the piece, my job was to give corrections when dancers did something wrong. Once I worked out the movement on the dancers, I relied on them to remember the choreography from one rehearsal to the next. The members, in turn, taught the material to others, while I focused on clarifying instructions for movement quality once the performers had learned the steps. Though I had directed the choreography, I had not absorbed the dance in my own body. I myself had never danced the piece.

I created the work with the intention of using as much of the preexisting material as the dancers remembered, while drawing on Club O' Noodles's ethos of inclusion. As a result, I had created a dance using vocabulary and structures that departed from my aesthetic interests as a choreographer. This made me nervous about my ability to perform the choreography on such short notice. In other words, in my own mind, I had agreed to participate in the choreographic process under the aegis of research, believing that in providing an account of the process I could still produce an analysis of its structure and possibly of the choreography's representational intention. I believed this could happen in both the spatial and temporal distance between myself, as the choreographer, and the performers doing the performing; which is why, in the original choreographic process, I did not attempt to master (in my body) the choreography. The prospect of having to "do the dance" ruptured my carefully rationalized framework for narrating my role as "an increasingly participating observer who makes a dance as research."

From the perspective of dance research, performing is often thought to give the researcher access to intimate knowledge about the dance itself, revealing something about how the aesthetic, social, and philosophical elements of the dance relate to one another to create meaning. Performing a role that I had a hand in creating meant that I would have to instill in the role a layer of interpretation that may or may not have anything to do with the role as it was intended by the director of the work. It is true that all roles are interpreted by the performers; however, at the level of representation there is not necessarily a direct correlation between the performer's interpretation and a viewer's interpretation of the performer's interpretation.

The crisis of analysis caused by performing in the production proves useful in considering the relationship between form-as-intention and the actual bodily experience of performing. For example, in the name of inclusionary politics, improvisation was an important component of Club O' Noodles's work; however, inclusion did not mean that the work was easy or was less demanding to perform. The frequent use of improvisation required the performers to possess a tremendous amount of awareness and versatility. Pieces designed for ease of adaptation did not translate into pieces that were easy to perform.

This became evident while I prepared for my appearance in *Nail Salon*. As part of Club O' Noodles's ethic of inclusion, teaching someone a new role meant having extreme confidence that the learner will "get it," but a two-day lead time was an extreme case. Unlike *Laughter,* in which more experienced members could easily exchange roles while coaching/prompting new members in the wings between scenes, the material in *Nail Salon* was still relatively new to most of the cast. The members, even veterans of the East Coast production, were still struggling to remember and develop their own roles, so everyone was on their own once the performance began.

What follows is a reading of *Stories from a Nail Salon* that is informed by the multiple and fragmented positions from which I viewed the production. I watched the production from either backstage or onstage, but I never had the opportunity to watch the production live from beginning to end. The existing video documentation of the work features an edited version of the performance spliced together from four shows of the same run, but with slightly different casts. This is an ethnographic account of the performance, of seeing it incomplete and from a visibly obscured position that is both far removed from some of the material, while too close to other parts of it.

The Performance

Stories from a Nail Salon is about the dreams and fears of five manicurists (or nail technicians)—Moc, Hoa, Dat, Thuy, and Kim—who work together in a Vietnamese American–owned nail salon. Moc, a thirty-something artist, is the manager of the nail salon. Hoa is an elderly, divorced woman with grown children and a penchant for gambling at casinos in her free time. Dat is an elderly man who spends much of his time reminiscing about his former life as a soldier in the South Vietnamese army. Thuy, a young woman, moved across the country in order to escape an abusive family; and Kim is an illiterate, mixed-race (black and Vietnamese) man.

Most of the action takes place in the nail salon, represented by a fairly simple set design in which four chairs are placed in each quadrant of the stage, facing the audience. The nail technicians sit in chairs representing their stations, while Moc sits behind them on an elevated stool so that he can look down over them. Everyone wears a white lab coat, and a white dust mask covering mouth and nose; they each hold a fake rubber hand that has inch-long acrylic nails glued to the ends of the fingertips. A sound recording of continuous sanding accompanies the workers' actions as they file the nails, massage, and otherwise focus intently on the fake rubber hands, representing disembodied customers. Working in silence and dressed in identical white coats, with their facial features obscured by the white masks, the workers appear anonymous to their bodiless clients, to the audience, and to each other. The scene brings themes of silence, disembodiment, and distance between the workers—and between the workers and their clients—and foreshadows the conflict and alienation among people who live and work in close proximity. The workers' silence, accompanied by the constant sound of sanding, is punctuated by their arguments, which grow in intensity until Moc demands silence from everyone. At this point, the workers interrupt themselves to address their fake hands: "Oh, no, he's not yelling at you. What color would you like?"

GHOSTS

A ghostly figure (a seminude male covered in white body paint) enters the salon. The ghost sits or lies down next to each of the workers to signal the beginning of that worker's monologue. This ghostly figure represents the unconscious of each character, who projects his or her fears onto him. The first time the workers enter the nail salon in the morning, they find the ghostly apparition in the middle of the room and ask each other what this "thing" is doing there. Hoa sees the ghost as a useless body, reminding her of family members who did not help her when she felt she needed it most. She calls the ghost a fat and lazy thing that looks a little like her ex-husband. Kim finds the ghost near his workstation and yells in Vietnamese, "My desk is not a trash can! Look at it!" The ghost stares back in his face and invokes memories of Kim's childhood. Kim imagines that the ghostly body is someone from his past mocking him and calling him "bastard." Thuy sees the ghost as a child frightened by abusive parents and she rushes over to protect it from Kim.

The performance locates the nail salon within the elusive nature of the American Dream. Each character has chosen to work in a nail salon in order to chase her or his own vision of freedom; but the work turns out to be mind-numbing and the five people pass the bulk of their day bickering with one another in Vietnamese, all the while working on the hands and feet of their Anglo and African American clientele. Throughout the performance, the actors lapse into bickering so frequently that the constant squabbling functions as a white-noise background, in which individual voices go unnoticed. It represents the degree to which each character is alienated from his or her own aspirations, family, and each other. The performance alternates between scenes depicting individuals' psychic struggles and the collective consumption of Hollywood films and *Paris by Night* videos (Vietnamese-language variety shows) to provide relief from the monotony of working in a nail salon and escape from personal demons, disappointments, and traumas.

As in *Laughter*, Club O' Noodles makes liberal use of popular culture in *Nail Salon*; however, its engagement differs in the latter work in that it examines a Vietnamese American desire for popular culture perceived as "better" alternative narratives to reality. In *Laughter*, Club O' Noodles aimed its comedic critiques at mainstream representations of the Vietnam War that relegated Vietnamese and Vietnamese Americans to a handful of recycled Orientalist stereotypes. In *Nail Salon*, Club O' Noodles drew both on Hollywood romances that, on the surface, have very little to do with Vietnamese Americans, and on Vietnamese-language variety shows featuring dancers lip-synching to Vietnamese renditions of American pop songs. One could say of the latter—produced and performed by Vietnamese people in Vietnamese —that they are products of self-representation and thus Vietnamese immigrant consumption of them constitutes an empowering act. *Nail Salon* critiques Vietnamese American consumption of popular culture as a form of escape and denial.

TITANIC AND THE POPULAR CULTURE QUEEN

In *Nail Salon*, Club O' Noodles uses references to popular culture to present community in conflict—in this case, the five workers. For Thuy, the blockbuster film *Titanic* is a romantic fantasy; but for others, the film triggers nightmarish memories of the one million Vietnamese refugees who died at sea trying to escape from Vietnam after the fall of Saigon. From her station, Thuy asks her co-workers: "Have you seen the movie *Titanic*? It was so good. I cried so much. I want to be just like Rose, and have someone sketch me." She gestures toward her neck and recites dialogue from the film: "Wearing this, wearing only this."

Annoyed, the older workers dismiss and chastise her for her obsession with the film, but Thuy ignores their comments and asks Kim to change the channel on his television so that she can watch the Oscars. Kim tells her no, because "all they do is talk," and Kim does not understand English. Kim wants to watch his *Paris by Night* video and eat his food; Moc intercedes and orders Kim to attend to a customer who has just walked into the nail salon. Kim shoots back at Moc, "I haven't eaten anything all day!" Moc ignores him and Kim transforms into the anonymous Vietnamese nail salon worker as he quietly puts his food away, puts on his mask, and politely greets another rubber hand.

Moc leads another customer to Dat, but the customer does not want a man to work on her hands. Moc then brings a male client to Dat, but Dat refuses to work on a man's hands and argues with Moc in front of the customer. (The customer is represented through gesture aimed at a rubber hand.) Time passes. When the last customer leaves, Thuy takes the opportunity to ask everyone if they want to watch television or go to the movie theater to see *Titanic* again with her. Dat wants to know why she and the rest of the country are so obsessed with the movie. He wants to know what about it people think is so good. Angrily, Hoa interrupts, "Nothing. It's about all these people who died on a boat." Despite Dat's and Hoa's attempts to dampen her enthusiasm, Thuy's face lights up and, with a dreamy look on her face, she proclaims that the movie looks so real and the story is so sad. To which Hoa replies, "So what? Who cry for the boat people? They die too. In many boats." The pace and volume of the bickering pick up until Kim, who has been trying to watch his television program, gets frustrated and yells above the commotion, "Forget it, everyone. Let's all just go and watch the *Titanic*."

Everyone exits the stage and a voiceover announces: "A little to the left. Slow it down. Now to the right—not too fast. Careful. What's that over there? Let's get a closer look." The actor who plays The Ghost (also known as The Unconscious) reappears as a faint image in the background. A giant screen made of newspapers glued together at the edges hangs down from the rafters in the ceiling. The newspaper is translucent: an image projected onto the back of the screen is visible to the audience sitting on the other side. Behind the newspaper screen is The Ghost, who is standing over an overhead projector, which illuminates his face. The light from the projector is bright enough to illuminate the space behind the screen also, thus doubling the size of the stage that the audience sees in the scene. The Ghost draws a figure of a woman, which is projected onto the back of the newspaper screen.

As The Ghost continues to draw, a voiceover says, "Is that what I think it is? Oh my God! I think we've found it. It's the Heart of the Sea!" and is followed by a steady pinging. Thuy reappears from upstage left and Kim chases after her in a melodramatic, one-minute reenactment of highlights from *Titanic*. Thuy stands up on a chair and spreads out her arms, while Kim holds her around the waist from behind. Thuy says, "Jack, Jack, look, I'm flying," and Kim responds by clearing his throat and spitting. From offstage someone yells, "Watch out—iceberg!" which is followed by the sound of crashing waves and the loud crack of a ship's hull breaking in two. A few of the other performers roll and stumble onto the stage; each finds a chair to grab then rolls off stage, as if being washed overboard. Kim says to Thuy, "Rose, Rose, promise me that whatever you do . . . promise me that you'll never let go." Thuy looks at Kim and says, "I promise, I'll never go." Kim pleads, "Promise me. Never let go," as he slips away, sinking into the sea. Thuy cries, "I promise, I'll never let go."

Thuy and Kim exit the stage as Deline Cion, a Vietnamese Celine Dion impersonator, appears upstage left. Dressed in a red velvet *qipao* complete with a silver phoenix appliquéd down the front and a six-foot-long gold Christmas tree garland draped around her shoulders, Deline makes a grand entrance. She lip-syncs to the soundtrack of a Vietnamese-language cover version of "My Heart Will Go On"—the theme song from *Titanic,* originally sung by French Canadian pop star Celine Dion. Dat enters the stage holding a fake plastic hand, just as Deline struggles to hit a high note. Flailing his arms about, Dat shouts, "I'm the king of the world." He then asks all television viewers to pause for a moment of silence and remember those who died on the *Titanic*'s disastrous voyage. The lights dim and everyone leaves the stage.

The rapid-fire succession of references to the boat people, the ghost of the dead, the *Titanic,* and Celine Dion is like a game of free association in which all are inextricably linked to the common theme of death and the sea. For Hoa, the racialized deaths of Vietnamese refugees is always under the skin of *Titanic*. If Hoa, forever haunted by memories of loved ones lost at sea, finds her memories in constant competition with Thuy's desire for a palatably romanticized vision of death, Deline Cion represents the nexus of memory and denial.

Deline Cion is clearly supposed to be a parody of *Paris by Night* videos. But why is she supposed to be funny? What is the audience supposed to see in her? The critique of Thuy's obsession with *Titanic* centers on the spectacle of memorializing disaster and the politics of who get memorialized. In this case, the fifteen hundred victims of the *Titanic* are memorialized as victims not only of a major disaster, but one that is domesticated as a unifying U.S.

tragedy. The southern and Eastern European immigrants traveling in steerage are folded into the "melting pot" narrative of early-twentieth-century U.S. immigration and sit comfortably within the matrix of U.S. history, which considers European immigration as the definitive descriptor of America as "a nation of immigrants." But the critique is not only about the implied politics surrounding the *Titanic,* but Thuy's inability to see what Hoa and Dat see in the film: a painful reminder of the way in which Vietnamese boat people are forgotten and would never be memorialized in such a glamorized and endearing manner. Deline Cion functions as an intermediary between Thuy, who wants to be Rose, and Kim, whose access to Vietnamese-language entertainment is mediated by a song from a film that Hoa and Dat find painful to watch.

I played the role of Deline Cion during the second weekend of the run. How should one play her? Is she supposed to be a "bad copy"? Do I make fun of the *Paris by Night* videos, which the members of Club O' Noodles constantly referred to as the genre they struggled to wean their Vietnamese American audiences away from in order to bring people into the theater where "real" and thought-provoking art is made? Is she supposed to be a bad copy of the bad copy? Or is she supposed to be a good copy of the bad copy? Or maybe Deline Cion is not a bad copy at all? Maybe the framing of Deline as a bad copy is really about the racist assumption that Asian bodies performing (Western or Westernized) popular cultural forms can only result in bad copies or copies period?

The performer who played the role the first weekend opted for an elegant diva whose lip sync corresponded to every lyric in the recorded music. She is the ideal object of Kim's nostalgic desire for Vietnamese-ness, as well as the key that allows him to participate in an aura of American culture from which he is linguistically other. This first Deline Cion could also be read as a translation of Thuy's Rose. Thuy can never be a white woman cast in the role of Rose, but Deline Cion marks the Vietnamese equivalent. Celine Dion's song, like most theme songs, operates like third-person narration. Closely associated with and aurally central to the film, the theme song still has a life of its own outside the film. Whereas Thuy's reenactment of the movie's love scene between Jack and Rose can only be read as a melodramatic parody, hearing a cover of "My Heart Will Go On" in Vietnamese is like hearing a dubbed film. Linguistically translated, Deline Cion is clearly marked as the best Asian copy who can sound melodically like Celine Dion, but is in no way mistaken for the "real" thing. Because she sings (lip syncs) in Vietnamese, Deline Cion does not sound *literally* like an English-speaking, French Canadian, white superstar.

Since I did not have time to learn the words to the song, I purposefully mismatched my facial gestures to the song lyrics. I chose to play the bad copy. My Deline Cion overperformed a poorly coordinated lip sync. If the other Deline could be described as smooth, regal, and aloof, mine was melodramatic and clumsy.

When Deline Cion's number ends, Moc enters the stage by himself. Alone and looking contemplative, he moves downstage toward the audience. He looks around the stage in silence until the sound of footsteps in soft, crunchy snow comes over the speakers. Moc reaches his hand into his pocket and pulls out a letter. Slowly and deliberately, he unfolds the letter and begins to read it out loud to himself in Vietnamese, while a voiceover provides a simultaneous translation in English.

"My Life and the Sea." The letter is written to Moc. The writer reflects on a series of memories, emotions, and dreamscapes stirred up while watching the film *Titanic* win a string of Oscar awards. Likening the sinking of the *Titanic* to the drowning of Vietnamese boat people, the writer is both Moc and not Moc, remembering family members and others who did not survive their escape from Vietnam. As Moc continues to read, the rest of the cast stands behind the newspaper screen. Reaching their arms and hands through slits cut in the newspaper, they change the spatial orientation of the stage. From the audience's perspective, the backdrop, lit with a dim blue light, becomes an ocean seen from a bird's-eye view. In the semidarkness, one can barely make out the outline of disembodied arms and outstretched hands and fingers—the final vestiges of people drowning at sea. As the last fingertips sink into the ocean, disappearing from sight, Moc finishes his letter to the sound of lapping water, and leaves the stage.

A woman's voice narrates a poem titled "My Life and the Sea," while the cast emerges from behind the screen and spreads out onto the floor from stage right and left. In pairs and trios, the cast "body surfs" across the stage by rolling over and under one another. The rest of the dance draws on a few simple movement actions reflecting images associated with water and the ocean: seabirds standing on one leg with wings outstretched; diving down into the water; rolling waves; and driftwood on a beach. Performers spread out across the stage and execute a movement phrase once through in unison. The phrase is made up of five movement motifs and gestures, upon which the performers improvise on their own, doing the movements in a different order and changing the timing and attack of each movement. After the improvisation, they move toward each other until they are all in the center of the stage, standing in a tightly knit circle. Each person then lunges and slides onto the floor, away from the center of the circle, followed by a quick recovery to a standing position. Using their own timing, the performers repeat their falling and standing sequence to create the effect of bodies tumbling out of a boat. Finally, everyone remains still, like pieces of drift-wood scattered on a beach.

Americana. This moment of eerie calm is interrupted by a sudden and spir-ited rendition of "Stars and Stripes Forever" blaring over the loudspeakers. Three people, each carrying a slide projector, walk across the front of the stage, projecting images onto the newspaper screen. The performers move so that they project a collage of images that moves in time with the music. Each performer has the same set of images, which he or she moves so that either three images or one distorted image is projected onto the screen. The first set of images consists of the Statue of Liberty, McDonald's golden arches, and the Vietnam War Memorial. These icons of nationalistic and branded main-stream culture are followed by more generic images of a school, a graduation, a new car. The last image features a grand opening of a new nail salon, finally marking a specific Vietnamese American subject.

The choreography of the slide show plays with the concept of distortion and the shifts between official national culture, the American Dream, and the reality of racialized labor. Each set of images is visually distorted as the performers move the projectors too close and too far away from the screen on which the images are projected. Occasionally, the three performers bring the slides into focus and create one single image that is recognizable before the image dissolves into the next permutation of American-ness. The focused and recognizable images are always fleeting, as they are quickly distorted and rendered unrecognizable—like the promise of the American Dream. The slide sequence takes its cue from the American Dream sequence in *Miss*

Saigon when The Engineer offers the audience a look into his fantasy of reestablishing his career as a pimp in the United States. The Engineer's fantasy ends with him riding in a Cadillac with Miss Chinatown sitting next to him, while a slide show featuring a number of iconic images (John Wayne, Marilyn Monroe, Betty Boop, New York City, Las Vegas, and, finally, bags of money) flash on a screen above the tableau. In the eyes of The Engineer, the United States is essentially an endless supply of economic opportunity linked to sexual excess.[2]

The American Dream in *Nail Salon* is far from glamorous. The symbols of citizenship (Statue of Liberty), global capitalism (McDonald's), and war (the Vietnam War Memorial) are followed by the markers of middle-class suburban aspirations (a college education and a new car). Desire for a college education and a new car cuts across racial, ethnic, and national boundaries, yet its placement in the performance also racially marks it as a particularized model-minority endeavor. With the images culminating in a slide of a nail salon, the road to the American Dream is shown to be decidedly unglamorous. The clean, sharp image of a nondescript pink-and-white, boxy stucco building standing in the blinding light of a hot Southern California sun belies any suggestion that what goes on inside can possibly be as glamorous as perfectly manicured, airbrushed, and bejeweled fingernails.

Like The Engineer's fantasy in *Miss Saigon*, *Nail Salon* includes its own Miss Chinatown. Representing a blueprint for ethnic Asian beauty pageants, Miss Chinatown is dressed exactly like Deline Cion as she leads a procession in a serpentine path around the stage. Like a mechanical doll, Miss Chinatown waves with her right arm and moves her head from side to side in a steady, rhythmic fashion, while the slide projections become increasingly distorted and out of focus until they are completely unrecognizable. Like the nail salon, Miss Chinatown, with her cheap dress, rhinestone tiara, gaudy boa, racially marked body, and suburban address, is not quite as glamorous as her televised counterpart, Miss America.

KIM

The rest of the performance is composed of a series of monologues, each told by a character who presents some aspect of his or her life story. All of the stories are imbued with a sense of longing—for closeness, the past, or a different future. The most striking aspect of *Nail Salon* is how it represents the invisibility of the nail salon workers via the literal absence of the customer's body. It is a portrait of an isolated world for workers who see no other employment opportunity. The fact that nail salons are associated with a luxury service makes them seem like unlikely places for labor exploitation. The performance gestures toward the way Asian labor is disembodied when the myth of the model minority stands in as the racialized version of the American Dream. Club O' Noodles manages to stage the invisibility of difference among Vietnamese Americans without obvious stereotypes to guide this particular representation.

For the rest of this analysis, I focus on a monologue titled "Kim" because it deals with the issue of mixed-race Vietnamese subjects. One of the underlying themes that informed the process of creating *Nail Salon* is the relationship between Vietnamese nail salon workers and their African American clientele. Although significant discussion regarding the economic dependence and reciprocal racism that occur between blacks and Vietnamese Americans within the environment of the nail salon happened during the rehearsal process, those discussions were not obviously integrated into the performance. Left out of the performance was the discussion of the practice of opening nail salons in or near neighborhoods with predominantly low-income black populations.

To a black female clientele, a Vietnamese nail salon worker might be an anonymous and interchangeably foreign subject who provides his/her service for half the price charged by white manicurists. Like Chinese laundrymen, cooks, and houseboys in the late nineteenth century, male Vietnamese nail technicians inhabit a feminized position. Masked and dressed identically, Vietnamese men are indistinguishable from their female coworkers. Reciprocating the racial stereotyping, a Vietnamese nail salon worker might view a black woman as someone on welfare who is nonetheless a source of steady income.[3]

For the most part, the conflict between black clientele and Vietnamese nail salon workers is invisible to the audience. One could read the complete absence of interaction between the nail technicians and the rubber hands as an overly literal performance of the lack of communication; however, I do think that would be an over-reading. Instead of dealing with the African American and the Vietnamese immigrant as discrete subjects, the performance includes a black Vietnamese character named Kim. Kim's story is based on that of an actual nail salon worker living in upstate New York who was abandoned at birth by his Vietnamese mother and African American father. Like many black Vietnamese children, he was ostracized in Vietnam and never sent to school by his adoptive family in Saigon. Illiterate in both Vietnamese and English, Kim worked in a nail salon staffed with other recent Vietnamese immigrants who would have considered him a pariah in Vietnam.

In the performance, the character of Kim is plagued by nightmares of Vietnamese children who hurl racial slurs at him. ("black dick, black ass," he tells us.) Sitting in a chair filing grotesquely long nails on a fake rubber hand, Kim alternates between making small talk with the rubber hand and telling the audience a tale of survival. He tells a story of a child who is a racial outcast, and starts hustling the audience in Vietnamese for food and money. Kim's body shrinks as he crouches close to the ground. He darts back and forth, hunched over, holding his hands out toward the audience, alternating between begging, cajoling, and insulting audience members. He returns to his seat and continues to file and stroke the rubber hand, while switching between light conversation directed at the hand and letting the audience in on his life as an illiterate adult trying to support his family as a manicurist. At unexpected moments, he is interrupted by the rest of the cast, who run onto the stage and encircle Kim. As though they were children taunting, the cast surrounding him chant "black dick, black ass." At the end of the scene, he states, "I don't regret anything."

In the performance, Kim is played by a Vietnamese American and does not "look black," begging the question of what a black Vietnamese person is supposed to look like. Kim's character functions as a significant intervention in the rubric of representations of blackness within the context of the Vietnam War. In the 1980s, the African American soldier in Hollywood film and the mixed-race Vietnamese orphan in the Broadway production of *Miss Saigon* cemented two representations of blackness in the context of the Vietnam War. Although African Americans made up a disproportionate percentage of troops sent to Vietnam, representations of the African American soldier in mainstream films are problematic. In Stanley Kubrik's *Full Metal Jacket*, for example, the infamous encounter between a Vietnamese prostitute and the African American soldier, which white soldiers observe with amusement, is based on foundational stereotypes of black men and Asian women.

In the scene, a Vietnamese man tries to pimp his sister to a group of U.S. soldiers; one of the black soldier takes him up on the offer. The Vietnamese woman vehemently protests and refuses to service the black soldier, and the pimp explains that his sister is afraid that the black soldier's penis will be too big. What follows is a predictable exchange, in which the size of black men's fabled large penises are celebrated and another round of financial negotiations finally convince the prostitute to have sex with the soldier. The systematic sexual exploitation of Asian women's bodies is projected onto the African American man, while the white narrator/soldier is represented as an innocent bystander, who can critically observe but does not physically participate in the sexual and political domination by the black soldier over the Asian woman and her brother. The Vietnamese man is pathetic and his sister easily raped; both are emblematic of Vietnam. The responsibility of the ridiculousness of the Vietnam War is placed in the hands of the black soldier, who stands in for the U.S. government. This film makes a very interesting narrative move, as the black soldier—who has barely left the Jim Crow South—is held visually responsible for the foibles of American foreign policy.

Kim's body is a projection of doubled stereotypes that African Americans and Asian Americans represent in regard to the conflicting representations of race and nationality. He is a foreign immigrant *and* a U.S. citizen in the absence of racial and cultural stereotypes that make visual sense to his body. Kim behaves like a Vietnamese immigrant, but he does not look entirely Asian. The blackness of his body provides the "evidence" that he is American and thus "owed" U.S. citizenship; however, Kim does not act like a "proper" American.[4] The failure of Kim's body to make visual sense is due to his body's excess of racial, cultural, and national signifiers. Invoking both absence and excess, Kim's story of complete rejection is unlike the stories of family reunions endemic to mainstream representations of the plight of postwar, mixed-race children left in Asia à la *Madama Butterfly* and the more recent *Miss Saigon*. Because Kim is not the child figure who can be theatrically saved by a white American family, the story of his adult life does not assuage American guilt over the Vietnam War.[5] Kim's body operates as a blind spot. In the performance, Kim's blackness is only addressed by Kim himself, in the form of the flashbacks that haunt him. His blackness is invisible to both his Vietnamese coworkers and the African American female clientele within the performance.

Overdetermining Community

Among the workers, Kim is figured as "more Vietnamese" than the rest of the characters. In this case, Vietnamese-ness is aligned with insularity and an obsession with money. Kim is the only one who insists on watching Vietnamese language videos, because he does not speak English. At the beginning of the performance, his inability to speak English appears to be unproblematically attributed to his immigrant status, echoing anti-immigrant sentiments that Asian immigrants do not assimilate.

While the other nail salon workers lament a former life (for them, nail salon work represents a dead end), Kim aspires to opening his own nail salon. In many ways, Kim's character embodies the overdetermined model minority. In an exchange with Hoa over the price of a manicure, Hoa describes her fellow Vietnamese nail salon workers as backstabbers who keep the price of manicures so low that no one can make a decent living. Kim thinks that Moc should lower prices or offer a two-for-one deal as a way to bring in more business. The clarity of Kim's biological claim for legal U.S. citizenship (his blackness or, more specifically, his other-than-Vietnamese-ness) is confounded by the ambiguity of what Vietnamese culture is.

Shaped by the forces of U.S. militarism, Kim's ambitions are the result of power imbalances created by U.S empire. The performance of *Nail Salon* does not couch its characterization of Vietnamese-ness (insularity and obsession with money) as cultural, but as a consequence of empire building and its relationship to immigration. In the context of the performance, Kim's position as a racial outcast in Vietnam heightens his abject position as a Vietnamese subject in the United States.

In this performance, there are no positivistic claims made about Vietnamese culture in regard to language, food, and customs. *Nail Salon* emphasizes the disaffection, distrust, and competition between a community of workers who do not see each other as a supportive network. At one point toward the end of the performance, Dat disappears and does not show up for work. None of the other workers knows what is going on with him, and no one displays any concern about where he is or whether something has happened to him. Moc simply tells the other workers to let Dat know that he is fired if he shows up to work late again. The seemingly insular space of the nail salon in its ethnic specificity does not offer its workers any more sense of belonging than does the "outside" world that ethnic-specific spaces are often set apart from. Momentary episodes coded as "Vietnamese American" dissolve, such that by the end of the performance there is no community in any positive sense; community simply becomes a matter of inhabiting the same physical space, without any emotional attachments. That Dat can simply disappear without his coworkers being concerned suggests the transience of what on the surface looks like a stable Vietnamese American institution.

If *Laughter* proposed a diversity of experiences that make up the Vietnamese American experience, *Nail Salon*—without a culturally affirming ending—proposes an absence of community. In *Nail Salon*, characters have no insights about each other's desires or fears, despite shared language, culture, and immigrant experiences. There is no affinity or affection between characters who, for the most part (aside from Kim), do not represent differentiated "types" in the way that those in *Laughter* do. *Nail Salon* engages with whiteness in such a way that it appears to have very little bearing or power over the workers' lives. Whiteness in the form of the film *Titanic* serves as a referent for unfulfilled dreams; however, the working conditions and how the workers treat each other happen in an isolated space. Even the clientele, rendered invisible, have little bearing on how the workers relate to each other. In many ways, the workers take each other for granted and see each other as transient and replaceable. There is nothing Vietnamese about the Vietnamese nail salon except the people who work there.

Conclusion

To consider the creative process in the reading of performance calls attention to the tensions within and between bodies—tensions that play out very differently in my accounts of The Popular Culture Queen and Kim's monologue. The analysis of the Popular Culture Queen, cast and recast at the last minute, sheds light on the work of performing. My reading of The Popular Culture Queen indicates the range of possible meanings offered by a performance structure that enables the performer to shape the role. However, the ability to shape a role does not necessarily result in a more informed interpretation of the representation, as evidenced by my not-quite-successful attempt to shift between the roles of performer and researcher. The shift between performer and researcher reads differently in my analysis of Kim's monologue. Written from a comfortable distance from the action on stage, the narrative unfolds like an objective account.

By attempting to integrate an account of the creative process in the analysis of a staged performance, my goal is to represent the extent to which the processes of creating and performing the work are rife with events that are not translated into the boundaries of the performance event itself. Discussion of the processes of choreographing, performing, and viewing performance makes visible the complex nature of accounting for the multiple ways in which writing about performance demands multiple embodiments. The body of the researcher, the performer, the viewer, and the writer is both whole and diffracted. In my discussion of choreographing The Popular Culture Queen and "My Life at Sea," the choreographic process focused on the formal elements of organizing bodies in space, much like the rhetoric of experimental performance and postmodern dance, which speaks of a body so present that one can attend to the metaphysical imaginings of the body's minute parts. In modern dance, dancerly talk often frames the ability to enjoy the wholeness of one's experience of the flesh-and-bone body within a language of fragmentation; for instance, the ability to zero in on and troubleshoot the placement of the right hip by lengthening the space between the top of the thigh and the bottom of the hip bone. This dancerly image of fragmentation in the service of the whole provides a useful methodology for framing the conflicting interests between the writing body, the dancing body, the viewing body, and the performance itself.

6

PEDAGOGY OF THE SCANTILY CLAD

Studying *Miss Saigon* in the Twenty-first Century

Summer 1996, New York City

After spending an entire day at the New York Public Library watching scratchy old videotapes of choreography by Mel Wong, Ruby Shang, Eleanor Yung, and the Asian American Dance Theater, I decided to go see *Miss Saigon*. Seven years after the first production of *Miss Saigon* premiered in London, I still had not seen the show that was billed as "A stunning piece of total theatre."[1] After reading countless editorials and academic essays about the casting controversy and racist stereotypes perpetuated by the production, I maintained my "Asian American activist" stance of boycotting *Miss Saigon*. But there I was, walking along Forty-second Street, seduced by the full impact of *Miss Saigon's* marketing campaign—the unavoidable glossy poster that beckoned to me wherever I went.

Besides, *Miss Saigon* figured prominently in *Laughter from the Children of War*, didn't it? I caved. I wanted to see what all the hoopla was about. I was staying at the home of a family friend, a well-educated and successful Asian American professional, who told me that he quite enjoyed *Miss Saigon* and he thought it unfortunate that some Asian Americans overreact and are too quick to protest "small issues."[2] So just how bad could it be, if an intelligent and cosmopolitan Asian American such as my host didn't think the show was as bad as Mary Suh (1990), Angela Pao (1992), Richard Fung (1993–94), James Moy (1993), Yoko Yoshikawa (1994), Dorinne Kondo (1997), and Karen Shimakawa (2002) had claimed it to be?[3]

Fascinated and distraught by my host's casual attitude toward a musical that had roused such passionate debate over sexualized racism, I purchased my $27.00 "half-price" ticket and sat in my seat in anticipation of seeing what the publicity had promised to be "total theatre." I laughed, I cried, I was moved, and my eyes filled with tears.

It is practically the end of the twentieth century and the best role my Filipina sister can get is that of a Vietnamese hooker. She does not have to wear the bad geisha-girl wig because she is a modern girl. No bell-shaped kimono for this sister. She gets to wear the Stars and Stripes in sequins pasted on her tits and ass. So, who cares if Mel Wong crossed racial and gender lines as the first Asian American man to dance in a major American dance company? You know, the one led by Merce Cunningham. You can see *Miss Saigon* really shake it six days a week, two shows a day, to sold-out crowds full of international tourists getting the big-city experience in New York, London, and wherever else this spectacle—of war and Asian female flesh—is exported by the touring company.

Spring 2000, Daly City, California

There is a Vietnamese restaurant in Daly City that I frequent on a weekly basis. I'm about to dig into a bowl of *pho* when I open up a copy of the *Manila Mail* and turn to an article about the anticipated September 30, 2000, opening of *Miss Saigon* in the Philippines.[4] Lea Salonga would reprise her role as Kim— an award-winning role that catapulted her career to international stardom. I chuckle to myself. How fitting that I am reading an article about *Miss Saigon* in the Philippines, reported in a Filipino American publication and distributed for free in a Vietnamese restaurant in Daly City. I continue eating and think back on the past year and the renewed popularity of Asian Americans in the news media. In 1999 alone, there was Wen Ho Lee, the Chinese spy that never was; hordes of anticommunist and anti–First Amendment Vietnamese American protestors who cannot seem to "get over" the Vietnam War; and, finally, Senator John McCain, whose "I hate gooks" comments did little to tarnish his image as a true American war hero.[5]

Spring 2001

Five hundred people participate in a March Against Hate rally at the University of Florida to protest a series of racist incidents on campus, including a fraternity party with an Asian theme. Fraternity brothers dressed up as

American GIs escorted women dressed up as Vietnamese prostitutes.[6] Imagine hearing the *Miss Saigon* overture in the background while assuming that the party organizers were not trying to offend Asian people. By the way, the Vietnam War and Vietnamese prostitution really did happen, right?

Fall 2004, Champaign, Illinois

According to my calendar, the touring cast of *Miss Saigon* is scheduled to perform at Assembly Hall on October 8, 2004, at the University of Illinois at Urbana-Champaign. Should I require all students taking Asian American cultural studies to see it? After all, Club O' Noodles created *Laughter from the Children of War* because of *Miss Saigon's* enduring popularity. Hung Nguyen explained, "I was standing outside the theater [after seeing *Miss Saigon* at the Ahmanson in Los Angeles] and this white man approached me and told me that he thought the show was so 'moving and beautiful.' [*pause*] I was horrified." This could be a good lesson plan.

Spring 2006, Montvale, New Jersey

For its world high-school premiere of *Miss Saigon*, St. Joseph Regional High School in Montvale, New Jersey, wins numerous awards at the Tenth Annual Drama Festival at Farleigh Dickinson University, at the Helen Hayes Theater Awards, and receives multiple nominations at the Paper Mill Playhouse Rising Star Awards.[7] By the spring of 2007, high school theater programs in Pittsburgh, Pennsylvania; Huntington Beach, California; Las Vegas, Nevada; and Chicago, Illinois, are staging their own productions of *Miss Saigon* as a lesson on the Vietnam War. The high school musical is not just entertainment—*it's a history lesson*. For many, it will mark the apex of theatrical aspirations; for others, the high school musical marks the beginning of a narrative in the pursuit of stardom.

Pedagogy of the Underdressed

I am sure some of you are asking, "Why another essay on *Miss Saigon*?" For one thing, Club O' Noodles's *Laughter from the Children of War* was created in response to the success of *Miss Saigon's* 1995 opening at the Ahmanson

Theatre in Los Angeles, and references to *Miss Saigon* have appeared in Alec Mapa's *I Remember Mapa*, Alison de la Cruz's *Sungka*, Maura Nguyen Donohue's *Lotus Blossom Itch*, and the 2005 Miss Saigon with the Wind Festival. *Miss Saigon,* as noted earlier, has been the subject of critical essays by Asian American theater scholars whose works address the intersection between the casting controversy and the problematic recycling of the Madame Butterfly narrative in the musical.[8]

Just two years after *Miss Saigon's* opening in Los Angeles, Dorinne Kondo described the energy and effects of the protests and casting controversies that occurred in New York, Minneapolis, and Los Angeles. Acknowledging the limited effect that the protests had on the production itself, Kondo emphasizes the significance of the publicity that the casting controversy drew to the production, calling it a "historical and political watershed that forced the mobilization of actors and community, spawning numerous artistic and political interventions that represent an array of tactical possibilities."[9] In spite of the protests, *Miss Saigon* remains one of the most popular musicals produced in regional and major theaters across the United States, Asia, and Europe, even though it closed on Broadway in 2001.

Miss Saigon's ever-growing popularity is a constant reminder of the marginal and perhaps even nonexistent space that performance art, modern dance, and dancetheater occupy in the public imagination. For artists like those in Club O' Noodles, coexisting with *Miss Saigon* is like sleeping next to an elephant. You can try to ignore it, give it room, attempt to push it away, claim to not mind it, but ultimately it will wake up and you will have to deal with the full force of its weight. Despite Club O' Noodles's efforts to stage a self-representative response, *Miss Saigon* has become so canonized in musical theater history that high schools and regional theaters proudly post video clips—of mostly white casts in various states of yellowface—performing scenes from the musical on YouTube.

To understand *Miss Saigon* as representative of the cultural forces that independent artists must continually work against, and to understand how it has managed to overcome its checkered past and become a musical theater "classic," this essay revisits the show almost a decade after its close on Broadway. Since *Miss Saigon* opened at London's Drury Theater in 1989, Asian American activists have been unsuccessful in their efforts to curtail audience support for the production's racially gendered stereotypes. Built on the bones of Puccini's *Madama Butterfly*, *Miss Saigon* features military uniforms and Asian prostitution—and represents a still racier fantasy. Written by two Frenchmen—composer Alain Boublil and librettist Claude-Michel Schönberg—*Miss Saigon* reduces U.S. wars in Asia to matters of circumstance and the supposed enemy state to a site of sexual fantasy. Nonetheless, the musical, performed in all major cities (and many small towns) in the United States and exported to Europe, Asia, and Australia, still operates as the most highly visible, successful, and economically viable performance featuring an Asian or Asian American cast.

The original discourse in support of *Miss Saigon* insisted that the musical manages to avoid a simplistic condemnation of the United States by focusing on postwar heroism in the form of sincere regret and charitable acts. In actuality, *Miss Saigon* represents the mainstreaming of white liberal antiwar sentiments as a revisionist history of Western imperialism. *Miss Saigon's* ingratiating representations of American characters engaged in charitable acts whip up emotional rather than political responses to the musical's antiwar stance. One is supposed to feel sorry for Vietnamese prostitutes, orphaned children, and U.S. soldiers—people who can be saved by love through marriage, adoption, and understanding. Marina Heung refers to this narrative structure as "the family romance," in which the prostitute, the orphan, and the soldier must form a nuclear family under the narrative logic of saving each other—the woman is saved from her degradation; the child, from poverty; and the soldier, from his guilt.[10]

Located outside this structure of family romance, the Vietnamese men in *Miss Saigon* cannot be integrated into the narrative of love because their interests lie in the realm of the political and the economic. If the military and sexual wrongdoings of the U.S. soldiers are made ambiguous in the musical, the military and economic interests of the Vietcong soldier and the pimp are clearly defined. Seeing the struggles of the woman, the child, and the soldier allows the spectator to participate in a collective feeling of sadness divorced from the racism and sexism of war and from politicized responses to those realities.

To deflect attention away from the musical's liberal use of Orientalist stereotypes, pro–*Miss Saigon* publicity maintains the musical's larger artistic goal by insisting upon war as the inevitable consequence of cultural misunderstanding. The framing of *Miss Saigon* as a study in cultural misunderstanding avoids a more explicit discussion of racism and of U.S. imperialism, thus shifting the focus onto white liberalism. This move creates the conditions for promulgating a mythic history in which the past is demonized as representative of bigotry and ignorance, while the present is celebrated as enlightenment and acceptance. The two time frames are distinctly separate eras in which one is a drastic improvement over the other. Present-day activists still arguing for social change are rendered extremists, since the big social battles have already been won. Overt discrimination is assumed dead; and when it does reemerge, discrimination is a singular act of tremendous ignorance and outside the boundaries of a mainstream United States that is fundamentally good, just, and well meaning.[11]

Miss Saigon's pedagogical reach extends beyond its claims for historical truth and social justice, and has functioned in the public imagination as a clearinghouse for aspiring Asian and Asian American actors, dancers, and singers for almost two decades. If the political aspirations of *Miss Saigon* are not enough to quell resistance to the musical's representations, *Miss Saigon* propaganda turns our attention toward the human element of the cast members themselves. Basically, if it were not for *Miss Saigon,* legions of Asian— and particularly Filipino—actors, singers, and dancers would go undiscovered and their Broadway dreams unfulfilled.

Supporters of *Miss Saigon* maintain its cultural validity as a necessary vehicle *for* Asian Americans, because it is the production in which one "proves" oneself before landing non-Asian roles. While *Miss Saigon* is credited with breeding an entire generation of Asian and Asian American talent, the plethora of new productions on Broadway featuring Asian or Asian American characters has not had the same impact. With the exception of David Henry Hwang's short-lived revival of *Flower Drum Song* (2001), *Miss Saigon* remains the primary employer for Asians and Asian Americans hoping to launch a career in musical theater.[12]

The Politics of Obviousness

That *Miss Saigon* has become a classic is a testament to what I call the "politics of obviousness." Its reach seems to include otherwise highly educated and culturally sophisticated individuals, including Asian Americans, who simply fail to see the musical's obvious stereotypes. As a semi-permanent tourist attraction in major cities all over the world, its continued success depends upon the marketing of the narrative as nonracist and "truthful."[13] The production not only provides a visual explosion of problematic constructions of racially gendered stereotypes linked to U.S. military activity in Asia, but it manages to breathe new life into timeworn stereotypes such that they are rationalized as "truer" and more accurate than previous incarnations. Even in the face of highly public protests by Asian American activists, the promotion of *Miss Saigon* centers around three arguments: (1) the musical subverts the very stereotypes that it deploys, (2) the musical implements a sophisticated critique of U.S. imperialism, and (3) the musical mines the depths of human tragedy. These rationales continue to sustain *Miss Saigon's* longevity.

After *Miss Saigon* closed on Broadway, the musical underwent what I consider a contextual transformation from cathartic Aristotelian spectacle to pedagogical resource. Its conversion resembles a kind of ideological appropriation of Asian American critique, such as found in the work of Club O' Noodles, given the self-referential content of *Miss Saigon's* publicity materials. This chapter revisits *Miss Saigon* to see how the production has managed to appropriate Asian American critique and transform otherwise obvious racial stereotypes into a neutralized educational documentary. The official *Miss Saigon* Web site, advertising the 2002–2004 North American tour by Big League Productions, includes a *"Miss Saigon" Study Guide* (Royston and Schlesinger, 2000) for teachers and educators to use in the classroom.[14] The format of the study guide is similar to those found on the Public Broadcasting Service Web site to accompany documentary videos and DVDs for sale to the general public. The *"Miss Saigon" Study Guide* refers to the reviews, souvenir books, and documentaries created to promote *Miss Saigon* as reference material about the Vietnam War; *Miss Saigon* is imagined as eliciting an entire realm of inquiry and a wealth of information.

The inclusion of the study guide on the *Miss Saigon* Web site suggests that the musical has not only transcended its troubled past (casting controversies and protests) but it has also transcended its status as entertaining musical theater. If, in 1991, the producers of *Miss Saigon* attempted to justify the production's sincerity and accuracy, the 2004 incarnation stands as an authoritative source of accurate information about the Vietnam War. The study guide foreshadows the entry of *Miss Saigon* into high school theater programs, in which directors cite the educational opportunity offered by the play when they are confronted with concerns about the show's racy numbers. Kathy Walter, a teacher at Spotlight Performing Arts Academy in Pittsburgh, Pennsylvania, viewed the school's 2007 production as "an opportunity for students to learn about a period in American History that is all-too-often ignored in history classes and textbooks." Walter explains,

> The cast most definitely feels the weight of telling a story as emotionally heart-wrenching and as historically significant as *Miss Saigon*. I want the students to take their work seriously and to be proud of their achievements. This is an opportunity for them to talk openly about what was a very troubling time in American history, and to be able to simultaneously reflect on current government policies and the effect that they are having worldwide.[15]

Describing the musical as "historically significant," Walter conflates narrative conventions and stock characters with history. Still, *Miss Saigon* serves not only as a lesson plan on the Vietnam War, but also as a source of information about war and foreign policy.

The study guide provides a synopsis of the musical's plot, followed by a series of suggested discussion topics and research/writing assignments on themes such as "culture and conflict," "lovers divided," and "the *bui doi*" (orphaned Amerasian children). Under the category of "culture and conflict," students are asked questions such as "What is culture?" and "Is it possible to have more than one culture within the same country? The same city? The same neighborhood?" Students are then asked to consider the effect of cultural clashes in everyday life, war, and ultimately how cultural differences and traditions between the East and the West are portrayed in *Miss Saigon*.[16]

These questions suggest that the production of *Miss Saigon* raises issues of cultural difference for the purpose of rectifying cultural misunderstanding; missing entirely are concepts of racism, empire, and power as driving forces behind war. Moreover, what is confusing about the study guide's focus on cultural misunderstanding is the fact that there are no real, consequential moments of misunderstanding in the show. All the characters understand perfectly well what is happening. One of the writing assignments asks the hypothetical student to consider how "Chris calls Vietnam 'A place full of

mystery that I never once understood'" (9). The guide proposes an assign-
ment in which students are instructed to, "choose a war (other than the war
in Vietnam), in which America has been involved, from the wars against the
American Indians to the Cold War with the Soviet Union" and asked to
"read about the conflict to discover how the opposing cultures differed" in
order to consider whether or not cultural awareness would have decreased
the likelihood of war (9). The focus on cultural misunderstanding displaces
the role of institutionalized racism that informs the production as a whole. It
blurs the distinction between history and Boublil and Schönberg's uncritical
reproduction of a nineteenth-century European fantasy (*Madama Butterfly*)
of interracial sexual encounter.

Guiding the viewer to see *Miss Saigon* as a tragedy and to ponder the
questions "Who is responsible for Kim's death?" and "By writing the ending
of *Miss Saigon* as they did, what do you think the authors were trying to say?"
the study guide diverts the viewer's attention from theater history and the
narrative conventions of the operatic tradition upon which *Miss Saigon* is
based. Modeled after *Madama Butterfly*, *Miss Saigon* reproduces all the key
narrative components of the libretto, such that Kim's death is a function of
narrative formula rather than a genuine mining of historical narratives.
Unlike *Madama Butterfly,* which features a long, drawn-out scene in which
Cio-Cio San's suicide is staged as an elaborate ritual, Kim simply goes into
her room and shoots herself without any real explanation or context. There is
no reason that Kim dies, other than the fact that Cio-Cio San always dies.

Complete with study guide and recommended readings, *Miss Saigon*'s
public image has moved from titillating spectacle to didactic documentary.
But there is a large gap between the current touring production, recast as an
educational reenactment of the fall of Saigon, and the anti–*Miss Saigon* protests of the 1990s chronicled by Esther Kim Lee. It is important to revisit how
the production has managed to overcome and repackage the troubled history
that followed the production in the 1990s. Between *Miss Saigon*'s London
premiere in 1989 and its 1991 opening on Broadway, debates over the controversial casting of Jonathan Pryce and, to a lesser extent, the problematic
representation of Asian characters in the musical were featured prominently
in the *New York Times*, the *Washington Post*, and the *Los Angeles Times*.[17]

Using the theatrical language of tragedy and melodrama as a metaphor for an already understood controversy, Jonathan Burton of the *Christian Science Monitor* writes, "Trouble over 'Miss Saigon,' the hit London musical slated for Broadway next spring, has kept anxious New York theatergoers and theater professionals on the edge of their seats for several weeks. Like the play itself, the dispute is tragic and melodramatic, combining race, money, power, and pathos." His article goes on to situate the importance of theatrical productions such as *Miss Saigon* within the economy of New York City, claiming that it could "easily pump as much as $100 million into New York's economy for every year it runs." Although Burton does not dwell on the casting controversy or the problematic narrative itself, both issues are referenced in passing as part of an assumed collective consciousness about what constitutes *Miss Saigon*'s "troubles."[18]

By 2005, any signs of *Miss Saigon*'s troubled past were entirely absent from reviews of the numerous reincarnations of the production. In place of references to *Miss Saigon*'s notoriety is language that institutionalizes the play's position within the theatrical canon as a Broadway classic. Any mention made of its past focuses on its success. Joe Piedrafite's review of the production at the Mullins Center in Amherst, Massachusetts, simply states that the musical "was one of the most expensive musicals ever produced, and it was also one of the most successful. Before it opened in the spring of 1991, it had an unprecedented advance sale, with prime seats going for $100, the top ticket price on Broadway at the time."[19] A 2005 review of the production in Binghamton, New York, situates *Miss Saigon* within a *Madama Butterfly* genealogy that begins with Loti's 1887 *Madame Chrysanthemum* and ends with David Henry Hwang's *M. Butterfly,* but fails to recognize the significance of its simultaneous presence on Broadway with Hwang's theatrical critique of the very narrative that the two productions share. Instead, the writer focuses on the success of its realism. "It's the sixth-longest running Broadway musical of all time, perhaps driven in part by the intensity of the dramatization of the evacuation of Saigon. Eymard Cabling, who plays the role of the Engineer in the touring production, said that moment, the famous 'helicopter scene,' captivates audiences" (Miller, 2005).

In his 1991 review of the Broadway production for *Time,* William Henry foreshadowed the political cleansing of *Miss Saigon,* musing about the day that it would finally be enjoyed as "just entertainment."

If spectators can clear their minds of the hoopla about the record $37 million advance sales, the $10 million production cost, the $100 top ticket price, the ethnic controversies over stereotypes and casting, and the residual political furor over the Vietnam War—in other words, of all the things that make *Miss Saigon* an event rather than simply an entertainment—they may find that the musical opened on Broadway last week is a cracking good show. It blends a love story and a spectacle with tragic social commentary about what the West symbolizes to the Third World, which is not peace and freedom so much as money and security.[20]

If only *Miss Saigon* can be seen without the political debates, then, finally, *Miss Saigon* can exist as that "cracking good show" that deals with "geopolitical rescue missions that turn into fiascoes, whole peoples' opportunities being thwarted through accidents of birth, the sheer randomness of how riches are distributed on this planet" (Henry, 91). In other words, *Miss Saigon* will ultimately be remembered as an artistically innovative and progressive production, once people can see it for what it is. And that is exactly what *Miss Saigon* has achieved fifteen years after its premiere. According to the Web site of the 2004 U.K. national tour (www.miss-saigon.com), the show had been seen by over thirty-one million people, translated into ten languages, performed by twenty-one companies in over nineteen different countries, and grossed over $1.5 billion.

Instead of an ever-present awareness of the "ethnic controversies over stereotypes and casting, and the residual political furor over the Vietnam War," the show is now followed by the quest for traces of the original *Miss Saigon*. These traces are found in such publications as the *"Miss Saigon" Study Guide*; Edward Behr and Mark Steyn's souvenir book, *The Story of "Miss Saigon"*; and David Wright's documentary film *The Making of "Miss Saigon."* The souvenir book (published in 1991 and now out of print) and the documentary are considered treasured "must-haves" by die-hard fans of *Miss Saigon*—the former more so, due to its out-of-print status.

The Story of "Miss Saigon," with its numerous color photos of the original cast featuring Lea Salonga and Jonathan Pryce, in tandem with the film *The Making of "Miss Saigon,"* documenting the competition between Lea Salonga and Monique Wilson for the lead role of Kim, offers *Miss Saigon* fans a memory of the original production, which can no longer be completely reproduced in its touring version. The real helicopter has been replaced by a video projection, and the worldwide quest for the perfect Kim is now filled by an ever-changing cast of Filipina women, none of whom has achieved the same level of international stardom as Lea Salonga.

Despite its much-touted out-of-print status, *The Story of "Miss Saigon"* is surprisingly easy to procure through Web sites like Amazon.com. *Miss Saigon* fan sites refer to it as both an important resource for accessing the original production and an insightful source of information about the Vietnam War itself. The questions posed in the study guide are also based on material presented in *The Story of "Miss Saigon,"* as if the souvenir book should be used as a textbook about the Vietnam War rather than as a document of the making and marketing of the musical.

Analysis of *The Story of "Miss Saigon"* demonstrates the logic of Henry's desire for *Miss Saigon* to one day overcome its troubles. Behr and Steyn present *Miss Saigon* to their readers as both a thoroughly researched production that accurately documents a dark moment in U.S. history, and as a musical that addresses universal themes of love and cultural misunderstanding. Framed as a serendipitous match of form to content, the translation of Puccini's operatic vision of nineteenth-century Japan into a musicalized rendition of the Vietnam War naturalizes *Miss Saigon*'s problematic representation of Asian women as harboring an affinity for prostitution and suicide. At the time of its publication in 1991, *The Story of "Miss Saigon"* was clearly a reaction to *Miss Saigon*'s "troubles," referred to in every review about the show. Fifteen years later, its contents had become a historical artifact, like *Miss Saigon* itself—such that the book, the show, and the study guide work together as a conceptually "perfect" lesson plan.

To revisit the opening paragraphs of this chapter, the answer is, "No, I did not end up making my class go see *Miss Saigon*." The $30 student ticket price played a key role in the decision. But, of course, I went. I remember sitting in the theater, just as I did back in 1996, counting off all the recycled stereotypes in the musical, and wondering if anyone could fail to recognize the production as an embarrassingly racist depiction of Vietnam and of Asian women in general. But it did not seem as if anyone else noticed the problematic representations, given the enthusiasm of the audience's standing ovation. This response served as a reminder that, even a decade after Club O' Noodles created *Laughter from the Children of War,* the work still speaks to the power with which *Miss Saigon* holds sway on the public consciousness. For this reason, it is crucial to revisit and examine the ways in which *Miss Saigon* is framed as high art, journalism, and antiwar activism.

Like the study guide, *The Story of "Miss Saigon"* includes an historical overview of the Vietnam War as well as an account of the writing, composing, casting, and rehearsal processes. Unlike the study guide, *The Story of "Miss Saigon"* includes a history of Orientalism in Western theater, as well as a chapter that relates the controversy and protest over the casting of a Caucasian actor in the role of The Engineer—a Eurasian pimp. Behr and Steyn package *Miss Saigon*'s recycled Madame Butterfly narrative as a matter of style. (I call it "style" for lack of a better word to describe the gap between the critique of *Butterfly*'s Orientalist theme and the "nonracist racism" used to justify its redeployment of stock stereotypes in *Miss Saigon*.)

Miss Saigon is Madama Butterfly

Miss Saigon is *Madama Butterfly* set in Vietnam, a fact that Behr and Steyn make no effort to hide. They make a concerted effort to place *Miss Saigon*'s adaptation of the *Butterfly* narrative within the lineage of opera in such a way that it does not simply inhabit the space of musical theater as middle-brow theatrical entertainment. Evoking Puccini elevates the form by aligning it with a classic of an elite Western stage tradition. Not only do the authors place *Miss Saigon* within the lineage of opera, but they also position it as an *improvement* over the historical development of Puccini's 1904 operatic adaptation of the Madame Butterfly narrative.

In "Butterflies to Bar-girls," Behr and Steyn provide a historical overview of the Butterfly motif, which has been the most enduring representation of Asia-as-woman since the exotic allure of Pierre Loti's autobiography, *Madame Chrysanthemum.*[21] They criticize the colonialist representations of Japan in Loti's book, which inspired Andre Messager's 1893 opera and John Long's 1898 short story "Madame Butterfly." David Belasco adapted Long's version for the stage in 1900, which in turn provided inspiration for Puccini's adaptation, now heralded as an artistic masterpiece.

[N]o other opera has ever recovered from such a violent opening night fiasco to earn so secure a place in the permanent repertoire. Puccini, Giacosa and Illica withdrew the piece, reworked it (giving Kate Pinkerton's song to Cio-Cio San, among other things) and emerged with a work which took the Chrysanthemum/Butterfly story to its apogee.[22]

Moving seamlessly between criticizing the trope and justifying its reappearance in *Miss Saigon,* Behr and Steyn recognize the Butterfly trope in Rogers and Hammerstein's *South Pacific* (1949) and *The King and I* (1951). They even go so far as to specify these productions' racist representations. Criticizing the golden era of musical theater and demonstrating their command of theater history, Behr and Steyn say, "[E]ven well meaning liberals like Hammerstein seem unable to make Oriental women anything other than passive non-characters."[23]

Following-up with a reference to David Henry Hwang's *M. Butterfly* (1988), which opened on Broadway one year before *Miss Saigon* opened in London's West End, Behr and Steyn align *Miss Saigon* politically with *M. Butterfly*. "In his play *M. Butterfly*, David Henry Hwang turned the myth on its head, showing how a shrewd Oriental could play to advantage a Westerner's need for a passive Butterfly."[24] They accomplish this via temporality:

Had he insisted on the story being told musically, the West End might have ended up with two musicals on the Butterfly theme side by side—the Hwang story and *Miss Saigon*. As it was, Hwang and his lead actor, B. D. Wong, were subsequently to cross Cameron Mackintosh's path in a way he could never have foreseen."[25]

Behr and Steyn seek to prove their intellectual capability by this brief analysis of *M. Butterfly*'s critique of Orientalism. Their championing of *M. Butterfly* and claim that *Miss Saigon* is like-minded make a case for *Miss Saigon* to be more like *M. Butterfly* than the "racist" representations put forth by Loti, Long, Belasco, Puccini, and Rogers and Hammerstein. In the end, however, Hwang and Wong (the playwright and star of *M. Butterfly,* respectively) are characterized as virulent proponents of censorship in their support of protest against the casting of Jonathan Pryce. In this manner, the writers align *Miss*

Saigon with *Madama Butterfly*, which serves another function—to justify the ultimate success of *Miss Saigon*. They cleverly allude to *Madama Butterfly*'s less-than-enthusiastic reception when the opera opened in La Scala in 1904; the opera suffered from bad press during its initial premiere, yet managed to survive. The authors frame *Miss Saigon's* public image as an omen that it is destined to outlive its critics and become a classic once the dust settles.

No longer a colonialist stereotype, Butterfly is recast by Behr and Steyn, with her demise resulting from a cultural gap between East and West reconstructed as "mutual misunderstanding."

> Instead, the name symbolizes the lengths to which the Americans, British and French—nations most seduced by *japonisme*—had to go to vanquish the real Japan. Some time after the atomic bomb was dropped, it was decided to erect a statue of Madame Butterfly in the town—on the estate of Tom Glover, the Scots merchant who introduced whisky to Japan and who, according to some, was the lover of the real-life Butterfly. In its complex intertwining of fiction and fact, this monument represents as well as anything the illusions which have so misled both East and West, and the yawning gulf which still separates the two cultures.[26]

They forget that *Madama Butterfly* was not based on a grand misunderstanding, but on a conscious attempt to create a fantasyland to entertain Western audiences. By suspending reality, Belasco and Puccini created believable fairytales. Behr and Steyn spend an entire chapter criticizing *Madama Butterfly* then proceed to ignore their own in-depth analysis in order to recount how *Miss Saigon* is a celebration of an artistically brilliant, yet racist, legacy. Racism becomes an unfortunate side effect of the Madame Butterfly narrative, rather than the reason for the stereotype's existence and continuing success. Orientalism is recast as a love story in which boy meets girl, boy loses girl, girl gives up child, and girl kills herself. From this perspective Boublil and Schönberg have improved upon *Madama Butterfly* by removing its racist elements, which they consider cosmetic rather than structural, and creating a formulaic tale of missed opportunities.

The study guide manages to avoid the issue of racism in *Madama Butterfly* by briefly mentioning that *Miss Saigon* "was inspired by a 95-year-old tale of Asian American romance that began with the publication of a story by John Luther Long called 'Madame Butterfly' in *Century Magazine* in 1887" (Royston and Schlesinger, 10). The guide does not provide any other information about "Madame Butterfly," except that it is a story emblematic of "lovers divided by race, nationality or religion" and that such stories (frequently?) appear in literature and drama (10). One cannot help but notice that the choice of terminology—"Asian American"—to describe Long's "Madame Butterfly" is paradoxical.

Miss Saigon's librettist, Alain Boublil, tells of coming across a photo of a Vietnamese mother parting with her child at Tan Son Nhut Airport and of identifying her as Madame Butterfly. This narrative is mythologized in *The Story of "Miss Saigon."* The study guide identifies this incident as the source of Boublil's inspiration; however, it does not acknowledge that the woman is a Madame Butterfly character. Instead, she simply represents pain and courage, and the authors make no mention of *Miss Saigon*'s relationship to *Madame Butterfly*. Self-contained and without reference to a theatrical or operatic genealogy, *Miss Saigon* becomes a historical document in the pedagogical process.

The fact of Madame Butterfly as a pervasive theatrical trope is essentially ignored in the study guide, as revealed in a lesson on how to "create your own musical." Readers are instructed to "select a photograph (from a newspaper, magazine, or textbook) that makes a powerful statement to you" and create a musical based on stories inspired by the photograph (Royston and Schlesinger, 13). The lesson plan is a familiar exercise taught in introductory acting or playwriting classes. The study guide's failure to fully account for *Miss Saigon*'s indebtedness to *Madama Butterfly* aids the documentary, *The Story of "Miss Saigon,"* in constructing the mythic origins of *Miss Saigon*, whereby Boublil "discovers" the original "Miss Saigon"—the actual woman herself. Boublil's problematic identification of the original Miss Saigon is parsed down to a lesson on the formal elements of the musical, such that *Miss Saigon* can serve as a universal example of how to structure a creative process.

The retelling of Boublil's discovery becomes a creation myth in which Boublil experiences a singular and visceral moment of inspiration that marks a gut reaction.

I was so appalled by the image of this deliberate ripping apart that I had to sit down and catch my breath. I suffered for the mother as though I might see my own little boy leaving me forever and I suffered for the child as though in my early youth had I been forcibly removed from my parents. Was that not the most moving, the most staggering example of the 'The Ultimate Sacrifice', as undergone by Cio-Cio San in 'Madame Butterfly,' giving her life for her child?[27]

Using the language of bodily instinct, Boublil naturalizes the association of the woman in the photo with Madame Butterfly's fate. Marina Heung attributes the centrality of the photograph's placement within *Miss Saigon*'s mythic origins as a result of Boublil's lack of imagination, because *Madama Butterfly* is what she calls the "foundational narrative of East/West relations" and a "master-text of Orientalism."[28] Given this logic, Boublil can think of the Asian woman only as a Madame Butterfly, and seemingly without being aware of it.

What remains baffling is the transformation of Boublil's parental empathy into the actual staged representation of the woman. Boublil empathizes: "She knew, as only a woman could, that beyond this departure there was both a new life for her daughter and no life at all for her, and that she had willed it."[29] Yet, on stage, this empathy is clouded by a fantasy of transnational interracial couplings coded as both tragic and dramatic. Boublil translates the middle-aged woman in the photo, whose face is drawn and weathered, into a highly sexualized stripper in his libretto. Translated again, the woman, clearly alive in the photo, is metonymically dead within *Madama Butterfly* as a meta-narrative. Projecting into the future reality beyond the moment caught in the photograph, Boublil cannot imagine that a Vietnamese woman can expect anything more than a racially stereotyped suicide.

Boublil's reaction seems to imply that all Asian women who enter interracial relationships are doomed to relive Madame Butterfly's fate. This is particularly disturbing because Madame Butterfly is a specifically racialized model of motherhood normalized to represent Asian womanhood. There is no evidence that giving a child up for adoption is racially specific to Asian women, nor is there any indication that the woman in the photo is heartsick over a lover. Yet, for Boublil, the Vietnamese woman in the photo can only imagine herself as a dead or a might-as-well-be-dead Butterfly.

Boublil's instant recognition of the woman in the photo as Madame Butterfly and Schönberg's twenty-year-old memories of Vietnam War news

footage represent their claim to profound artistic inspiration. They pat themselves on the back: "Like all really inspired ideas, *Miss Saigon* seems obvious
when you see it in its finished form: Madame Butterfly updated to Vietnam;
why didn't anybody think of that before?"[30] Somehow, inspiration coupled
with reawakened antiwar sensibilities, empathy, and memory is translated
into a production that borrows nineteenth-century Oriental stereotypes ab-
sented of Orientalism.

> Yet, by any standards, this was a writing assignment which pre-
> sented all manner of obstacles. "Pierre Loti's original book is terri-
> ble," says Schönberg of *Miss Saigon*'s source material. "It's a book of
> the nineteenth century, written at the height of European coloniza-
> tion. The character of Pinkerton is awful: she is a toy for him, so,
> when he comes back to the country with his American wife, it is only
> to pick up the child. There is no problem for him. So we took the
> basic story of 'Butterfly' and, considering that we were writing for
> 1989, tried to improve the human aspect. We didn't want Chris to be
> a bastard like Pinkerton—using a girl, leaving her, then coming
> back. So we changed the story completely—the way they did when
> 'Romeo and Juliet' became 'West Side Story.'"[31]

Boublil locates *Madama Butterfly*'s problematic representation in the character of Pinkerton, and "fixes" the Pinkerton problem by representing Chris in
a positive light. But this explanation of how Boublil reworked *Madama
Butterfly* fails to address the larger representational issue, in which the writers understand Asian women in nineteenth-century terms.

You'll Miss Saigon

Why should it be obvious that *Miss Saigon* should be *Madama Butterfly* set in
Vietnam? Why should audiences consider such obviousness a stroke of genius, when Madame Butterfly has been the predominant frame in which
Asian women have been depicted on the Western stage and in film for well
over one hundred years? Why continue the diatribe against such obvious
racism? In 1997, *Miss Saigon* represented just one of many musicals for which
tickets were on sale at any number of discount ticket booths in Times Square.

Rent, the upbeat musical about AIDS, took over as the hot new show in town and in the media. With its high-profile casting controversy quelled and its blatant racism explained away, *Miss Saigon* all but disappeared from the media. If one lived in California, without a Broadway theater district, it might seem as though *Miss Saigon* no longer existed.

But in the fall of 1999, I was shocked to discover advertisements for *Miss Saigon* all over London's subway stations. These advertisements did not use the familiar abstract, brush-painted helicopter image so well documented by the film *The Making of "Miss Saigon."* Instead, the new ads featured a color photograph of an Asian woman wearing an unbuttoned Army coat—with nothing on underneath. Above her head was the caption "You'll miss Saigon." The "clever" play on words, coupled with an unsubtle photograph, all but states that "Asia equals prostitution." After ten years, the production needed a new image to lure tourists into the theater, one that was more assertive in advertising what *Miss Saigon* promises to deliver.

The young woman in the photo leans against an object cropped out of the picture. She stares straight into the camera with her eyes half closed. Her expression is languid (or tired) and unsmiling. One side of her unbuttoned coat strategically covers her right breast, while a lock of her long hair barely covers her left breast. A wide, V-shaped expanse of flesh from her neck down to her waist is left visible, inferring that she is completely nude underneath. She is bra-less, but is she or isn't she wearing pants? We do not know, since the photo fades into darkness around her navel, suggesting that if we were to stand back far enough (maybe in the theater?), we would get to see more.

In the photo, she looks young; but just how young, we don't know. We assume that she is old enough that it is socially acceptable to look at her exposed cleavage. Unlike fashion photography, in which very young models are made up to look like mature adults, the "Miss Saigon" in the photo does not look as if she is wearing any makeup. Her unmade-up face connotes childlike innocence and naturalness. She looks vulnerable, as if her clothes are about to fall off any minute, and she is coded as a Vietnamese wartime whore. The combination of implied nudity and the military coat welcomes the viewer to see her as a racially foreign and sexually available commodity. Did she just turn a trick and slip on her client's jacket? Or is this her "look" when she's looking for new clients? This is what the musical is *really* about. It is no longer about the struggle over artistic freedom (casting controversy) or revolutionary special effects (life-size helicopter), but, rather, the promise of seeing a half-naked Asian girl-woman onstage.

Like the ubiquitous gongs and flutes that always accompany the entrance of an "Oriental character" in a television or film scene, *Miss Saigon* and its history are concretized as yet another stereotype that only needs to be referred to by name. It has managed to recede into a remote past, even as it continues to operate in the present. In 1993, Richard Fung called *Miss Saigon* an "interesting phenomenon" (7), but it is no longer a phenomenon. Now canonized, it has become a tourist attraction alongside *Cats*, *Les Miserables*, *Phantom of the Opera,* and a variety of other shows one can take in after a day of sightseeing in one's metropolis of choice. Without the hype of its earlier success and the intrigue and passions of the politically charged debates, *Miss Saigon* can take its time catering to a global population.

Clearly, the "obviousness" of *Miss Saigon*'s troubles can be rendered insignificant. William Henry's dream of the day when *Miss Saigon* can exist simply as a "cracking good show," sans the lowly politics in which Asian American protestors were mired, has come true. This dream is echoed in the rise-from-the-ashes narrative in *The Story of "Miss Saigon."* Like Henry's comment, Behr and Steyn's neutrally enlightened stance shores up charges of reverse discrimination leveled against the Actor's Equity Association (AEA) in 1991.

> An interesting aspect of the *Miss Saigon* protest was that the minority group raising the ethnicity issue was not black but Asian. What provoked the crisis was an awareness that the *New York Times*, in an important editorial, referred to as "a new tribalism, a heightened awareness of ethnic and racial separateness." The new trend, it said, was "in a proliferation of small cultures—an ethnic culture, a racial culture, a woman's, a gay's, a black's culture. Everybody seems to be looking at the world through the brightly coloured lens of his or her own particular group." This in turn, threatened to usher in a new era of conformity and sanctimoniousness.[32]

First, the logic employed in Behr and Steyn's comments is ludicrous: Why would one expect the black community within AEA to protest the casting of a white man in an Asian role?[33] In addition, surprise at the fact that Asians were bringing up the ethnicity issue—that it was not just "a black issue"—perpetuates the stereotypes of Asian Americans as silent and politically passive and of blacks as outspoken and politically active. Most importantly, these charges of reverse discrimination foreshadow a darker reality of racial discourse in the coming years. In 1996 the passage of the California Civil Rights Initiative (CCRI) banned affirmative action. Authors of the CCRI used the same tactical language of reverse discrimination to blame "the ethnics" for causing unnecessary racial divides in the United States.

Miss Saigon: It's Better Than You Think

I am constantly reminded about the "unobviousness" of *Miss Saigon*'s time-tested, formulaic strategies of representing Vietnam with a series of infantilized, effeminized, sexualized images. Using humor, Club O' Noodles's *Laughter from the Children of War* performs an undisguised critique of *Miss Saigon*'s aspirations for historical truth about the Vietnam War. In an interview, Tran confesses that, prior to joining Club O' Noodles, he had learned everything he knew about the Vietnam War from watching Hollywood films. Although it is not a Hollywood film, *Miss Saigon* has been marketed as a revolutionary theatrical work because it approaches the realism achieved by film.

Not only does Behr claim that *Miss Saigon* comes close to achieving a filmlike realism, but also that it surpasses the accuracy of Hollywood films about the Vietnam War: "With all this in mind, the opening number of *Miss Saigon* is for me far more convincing than almost any bar scene in the sixty-odd films that have been made about the Vietnam War."[34] He goes on to point out the multiple fictions about Vietnamese women perpetuated in the classic Vietnam War film *The Deer Hunter*:

> In particular the Tu Do street scene in *The Deer Hunter* (actually shot in Thailand) was far too frenzied, the sex too overt, the music too loud, the backdrop too luxurious. Even during the closing stages of the war, though bars and massage parlours were tolerated, their owners were cautioned to behave with discretion. In *The Deer Hunter*, a bar-girl go-go dancer takes Christopher Walken back to her tiny apartment and prepares to make love while her baby is awake and crying in the same room. Perhaps more than anything, this scene

reduced the film's credibility in the eyes of Vietnam veterans: they knew no Vietnamese woman would ever have made love to a customer in front of her baby.[35]

"The Saigon of *Miss Saigon*," the first chapter of *The Story of "Miss Saigon*," is written from Behr's point of view as a *Newsweek* war correspondent. In this chapter Behr sheepishly admits to having had sex with numerous Vietnamese prostitutes, an experience that allows him to vouch for the authenticity of *Miss Saigon's* representation of Vietnamese women. Behr's claim that he understands the true nature of Vietnamese women as innately modest, religious, and monogamous is framed within prostitution. Behr's Vietnamese women are prostitutes-in-waiting and his bar-girls are hookers with hearts of gold looking for real relationships.[36]

Popular representations of American military activity in Asia align prostitution with normative Asian female sexuality. Caricatures of the geisha girl, Suzie Wong, and the me-so-horny Vietnamese hooker fuel white fantasies of social docility and passivity, coupled with sexual promiscuity. By positing Asian women as "always already prostitutes," these images make Asian women the ideal sexual fantasy, since they, unlike white women, do not need to be incorporated into the American nuclear family. As victims of wartime circumstance and geographical distance, Asian women are easily killed off, left behind, or simply disappeared under the assertion of irreconcilable cultural difference. *Miss Saigon's* successful adaptation of a late-nineteenth-century European vision of Asia-as-female-prostitute is most disturbing, since the musical positions itself as a performance that is "not about the Vietnam War," yet also claims to be antiwar.

Miss Saigon as Antiwar Critique

What *The Story of "Miss Saigon"* would like the reader to believe is that its continuing success hinges on the premise that one is watching "intelligent theater" that is visually spectacular, emotionally riveting, and politically expedient. More bang for your buck if one can be entertained and "get" the musical's antiwar stance at the same time. The problematic love story inherent within the Madame Butterfly trope—and the formula that operatic heavyweight provides—is overwhelmed by *Miss Saigon's* alleged antiwar aspirations, backed up by advertising that focuses on its "authenticity" and supposedly revolutionary theatrical form. Mythologized as the ultimate form of art, the musical itself stands in as a substitute for diplomacy. It functions as a documentary that provides social commentary able to transcend national politics in order to deal with the one true, universal emotion—love. Behr and Steyn write:

> I believe that not only Kim, but also Chris, are believable characters. In real life, of course, they would have been less articulate. But within the framework of sung-through theatre, in what is an opera of the Nineties rather than a "musical," Alain Boublil and Claude-Michel Schönberg have invested them with the kind of truth we perceive in major classic operatic roles.[37]

Behr and Steyn rightfully claim that *Miss Saigon* does not aim to represent war, but significant attention is paid to building a repertoire of "truth" in regard to the *affects* of war. The "live" helicopter that lands onstage, the documentary-like slide show of abandoned *bui doi* children—which is not supposed to, but does, in fact, interrupt the narrative of the musical—and the "original" photograph of a Vietnamese woman saying goodbye to her Amerasian child have all become part of *Miss Saigon*'s cache of visual truths about the Vietnam War. These three images serve as evidence of the production's sincerity, which stands in as a panacea for American guilt and contributes to the ontology of the American soldier and the United States as victims of guilt. The French composer and librettist claim to have opposed the Vietnam War before American antiwar protesters did, and thus the legacy of French colonialism in Vietnam is relegated to a few French phrases quipped by the mixed-race French Vietnamese pimp in the musical. Despite the writers' vigilance as antiwar French citizens, the musical is very much in line with mainstream U.S. versions of the Vietnam War as a black hole for guilt.

Boublil and Schönberg's assertion that they came up with the idea of *Miss Saigon* before the release of the big Vietnam War blockbusters, such as Oliver Stone's *Platoon,* further bolsters the musical's claim to authenticity and originality. But aside from the costumes and focus on prostitution, *Miss Saigon* shares an underlying theme of guilt with films like *Platoon*. Framed as a uniquely American experience, the Vietnam War is an era for which Americans are unable to accept responsibility for imperialism, yet wallow in guilt over imperialism.[38] According to Behr and Steyn, even Richard Maltby Jr., one of the lyricists, succumbs to this: "Maltby at times seems almost the personal embodiment of American naïveté and guilt over Vietnam" (65). In Behr and Steyn's portrayal of *Miss Saigon* as a truly engaging work, the play's potential for controversy lies in its risky antiwar stance and not its racist representation of a Madame Butterfly narrative filled with requisite prostitutes, sneaky Orientals, white actors in yellowface, and a diabolical Oriental patriarchy from which the white man must save the Asian woman.[39]

The accessibility of popular representations of the Vietnam War reduces Vietnam itself to a war, absenting it of culture, language, and people. Instead, Vietnam has filled a psychic space in the U.S. imagination as a geographical expanse defined by a historical moment with no past and no future. It is an exotic and foreign location inhabited by dead or about-to-be-blown-away Vietcong, whores, oppressive jungles, and anonymous bodies dressed in black pajamas and conical hats, running around screaming unintelligibly. Liberal representations of the Vietnam War may also include a "critique" of war by showing wanton U.S. violence against Vietnamese women and children, but the antiwar sentiment is always embodied by an individual enlightened white soldier who is horrified by what he sees. If he is more liberal, he may also go as far as recognizing past wrongs and see the necessity for reuniting Amerasian orphans with American fathers.

Vietnam War as Interracial Prom

The subject of prostitution and the performance of prostitution is central to *Miss Saigon*'s configuration of Vietnamese women—something that the study guide reinforces. In section 7, "The War in Vietnam," the first suggested discussion question is, "How is Kim symbolic of the problems women suffer in wartime? Using the Vietnam Timeline, or your own research, think about what circumstance and events might have led Kim to become a bar-girl in Saigon and Bangkok."[40] This angle reinforces Behr and Steyn's assertion that *Miss Saigon* provides an accurate portrayal of Vietnamese women.

If *Madama Butterfly* has been aestheticized as a love story, decorated in the excesses of European Japanoiserie, then Behr and Steyn achieve distance from the original by criticizing it through strategic marketing. *Miss Saigon* is a love story of *Butterfly*'s proportions, with "a biting political message." But its claim to "truth," "authenticity," and "believability" should sound alarms. Behr fondly remembers the innocence of the Vietnamese bar-girls and prostitutes whom he admits to soliciting. He justifies his claim that *Miss Saigon*'s bar scenes are more accurate than those in Hollywood films, with his "been there, done that" credentials, which he puts to work in his reading of Vietnamese women through the lens of a cliché. Behr's firsthand account of Vietnamese prostitution reads like a teenager's first date.

> A discreet voyeur, I admired the girls' dexterity, circulating like fashionable hostesses at embassy receptions. Noticing each others' predicament, they would help their friends out, attracting the attention of the rival so he would not notice "his" girl and another man kissing. The GIs and bar-girls held hands a lot, and the necking and heavy petting that went on reminded me of the Fifties as I had vicariously experienced them in American movies.[41]

Behr reframes prostitution and an Orientalizing/fetishizing gaze within the language of "dating" in the 1950s (a period fabled to be more chaste than the turbulent '60s that he remembers).

It conjures images not of sexual exploitation, but of a boy-girl party, a school dance, and something that might be no more sordid than a high school prom—basically, a good time to be had by both American boys and Vietnamese girls. This nostalgic-1950s U.S. vision of prostitution becomes an appropriate premise for family entertainment, a prostitution emptied of the violence, disease, abuse, and humiliations suffered by the prostitutes themselves. From that perspective, prostitution is disassociated from the context of war—which is equally uncontextualized—and becomes a matter of interpersonal relationships rather than an institution driven by the pressures of economic underdevelopment and exploitative labor practices. Behr justifies prostitution as a necessary mechanism for white men to save Asian women (who are also innocent prostitutes) from Asian men.[42] Behr writes:

> A French TV documentary, made several years after the collapse of South Vietnam, showed some of these former bar-girls in "rehabilitation therapy," repeating, parrot-fashion, clichés about American

imperialism. The new Vietnamese authorities used these war victims to denounce their former "oppressors" in terms that were both
laughable and wildly inappropriate. Of course the whole bar-girl
phenomenon had been a by-product of the awful war, but this had
not prevented a form of warmth, or, in many cases, genuine relationships between the Americans far from home and young Vietnamese
women.[43]

Behr's logic insists that Vietnamese people have got it all wrong; perhaps
Vietnamese women were better off working as prostitutes and bar-girls.

In her study of sanctioned camp-town prostitution during the Korean
War, Katherine Moon documents the policies that formed part of the bargaining agreement for American soldiers to remain in Korea. U.S. military
officials routinely negotiated with Korean officials on health regulations for
prostitutes working in zones set up for the sole purpose of servicing U.S.
soldiers stationed in Korea. The U.S. military considered regular access to
institutionalized prostitution necessary for maintaining high morale among
U.S. troops during and after the Korean War.[44] This institutionalization of
military prostitution in Asia contextualizes Behr's account of the bar-girl
phenomenon so that it cannot be seen as an isolated instance of romantic
fervor, but as part of a systematic gender and racial hierarchy in which Asian
women are relegated to the role of sexual commodity.

Interestingly, when Behr does include a grim portrayal of Vietnamese
prostitution, it is in the service of dispersing the blame among the Americans,
Vietnamese, Chinese, and French. Such a fate renders prostitution relatively
benign. Behr considers the exploitation of Vietnamese female bodies by U.S.
soldiers "humane" and uses innocuous terminology to describe a typical
encounter between U.S. soldiers and Vietnamese prostitutes. Overtly sleazy
experiences are categorized as isolated horror stories that should not be
mistaken for what really happened to most Vietnamese women and girls.

The bar-girl phenomenon *was* regrettable, and the girls *were*, in a
sense, prostitutes, though even the "Gigis" among them, on whom
the hard-bitten, experienced girl in *Miss Saigon* is modeled, lacked
the haggard toughness of their Western counterparts [emphasis in
original]. And, of course, the exploitation, not only by Americans,

but by Vietnamese and Chinese entrepreneurs, functioning with the complicity of a predatory police force and military regime, was brutal. There were tales, too, of mothers selling their daughters, of Vietnamese "cowboys" seducing innocent girls and becoming their pimps. Outside Saigon, there were grimmer places, like the notorious garages where U.S. Army truck drivers could get their vehicles hosed down by Vietnamese soldiers while enjoying a "short time" upstairs with their girls. But the sex scene, in comparison with what it had been under the French rule (with the huge brothel complex, "Le Grand Monde") was less organised, and probably more innocent. The French had done things differently. Their colonial officials had picked out barely nubile orphans from religious institutions for domestic service and sexual enslavement, sometimes with the tacit connivance of the nuns themselves. "Le Grand Monde" apart, there had been officially run army brothels—Bordels Militaires de Campagne (BMCs)—in every large barracks, and some in the field—there was even one at the siege of Dien Bien Phu. In the final analysis, which form of exploitation was more humane?[45]

Behr romanticizes U.S. involvement in wartime prostitution to justify sexual exploitation as an institution that can save Vietnamese women from what they will suffer in the hands of another oppressor. Traise Yamamoto (1999) rephrased Gayatri Spivak's 1988 characterization of "white men saving brown women from brown men" as a project of "large-scale domestic intervention" or "pseudofeminism." Within this model of pseudofeminist gender equality, the West—embodied in the form of white men—becomes liberator, fighting against oppressive Asian gender hierarchies.[46] The Asian prostitute is the perfect victim, easily saved from the Asian enemy that the West is fighting against. Her body is literally a war reparation and, because her body is marked like the racially othered enemy, she must always die at the end of the story.

For this viewer, there remains a disconnect between seeing *Miss Saigon* in the theater and reading *The Story of "Miss Saigon"* or the study guide. From reading either text, one might imagine a staid and didactic production, not the overt display of sexually explicit lyrics accompanied by equally "dirty" dancing performed in a visually and aurally pleasing manner. The language of the study guide suggests that the show is age-appropriate for an elementary or junior high-school fieldtrip. It poses a series of questions to consider after watching *Miss Saigon*, such as "discuss how the war affects the lives of the following characters: Kim, Chris, The Engineer, Tam, Thuy," and asks students to consider "what kinds of devastating long term effects are felt by survivors on both sides of a war long after the conflict is over."[47] These questions underscore the assumption that *Miss Saigon* doubles as reference material on the experiences of people involved in the Vietnam War.

One hopes that a student who undertakes additional research would come across *Miss Saigon*'s troubled past and see clearly the musical's problematic reiteration of nineteenth-century stereotypes of Asia and Asian women. Contrary to the argument that *Miss Saigon*'s popularity can be attributed to its value as a pedagogical vehicle for teaching the public about cultural differences, the musical appeals to Western audiences because of its familiar movement vocabulary and singing.

Pedagogy of the Guilty

I return to the theatrical production in order to re-present a description of the two most visually important elements of the show, deployed to project a balanced program combining entertainment and the illusion of social consciousness. The Vietnamese bar-girls and the *bui doi* represent two ends of the guilt spectrum. Sandwiched between the woman and the child is the U.S. soldier, forming a triad of the victimized interracial family. *Miss Saigon*'s visual triangle of mother, father, and child mimics the structure of the nuclear family. In reality, the mother is a whore with no intimate loyalties, the father is a soldier sent to kill Vietnamese people (including women and children), and the child is an orphan. Vietnamese men are completely left out of this framework.

If the soldier experiences politics vis-à-vis the Vietcong, marked as male and chauvinistic, he experiences culture vis-à-vis the woman (in this case, a prostitute). To make a crude analogy: Vietnamese women perform Vietnamese culture—singing and dancing—for American men. Such a literal enactment of "culture"—the show within the show, featuring Vietnamese prostitutes at work—provides an opportunity to stage the "fun" part of the musical in order to temper the morality tale introduced by the slide show about the *bui doi*.

The production of *Miss Saigon* opens with that show within the show. After the lights come up onstage, a number of Vietnamese bar-girls/prostitutes, including a newly arrived Kim, complain in their dressing room. In various states of undress, the women sarcastically joke about the predictability of the evening about to unfold: "Tonight I will be Miss Saigon," "Tonight you will be Miss Jumped Upon." After a few more lines of cheeky lyrics while the women finish dressing, the stage set transforms into Dreamland, the quintessential Vietnamese girlie-bar. It is a place of rocking good times for American GIs, who buy raffle tickets in hopes of "winning" Miss Saigon—the winner of a nightly sham beauty pageant staged at the bar. The cast of American Marines, Vietnamese civilians, and South Vietnamese officers mingle in the bar; however, the song in that scene ("The Heat Is On in Saigon") is explicitly racist. The women are referred to as "slits"—a term that connotes racial difference, sexual pleasure, and derogation.

"Oh my God, did they really say *'slit'*?" screamed Joanne (a pseudonym) on the other end of the phone, after I read the opening lyrics to her. Along with "slant" and "slope," "slit" joins a list of derogatory *s*-terms regarding eye shape, used to identify Asian racial difference. Historically, the association between eye shape and Orientalness overrides skin color (Yamamoto, 1999). Yamamoto's analysis of the purported lack of an epicanthic fold as visual proof of Asian racial difference emphasizes the shifting category of "yellowness" in reference to Asians and Asian Americans. This is especially clear when one thinks about the extent to which Asians were legally racialized in the United States through a combination of differences around skin color. Yamamoto observes that Asians and Asian Americans as a racial group are invisible because they are rendered both racially different (as the yellow race) and not different (as "honorary whites") (63–64).

In order to prop up yellowness as a shade truly different from whiteness, eye shape is used to demarcate the undisputable site of Asian bodily difference.

> [F]rom grade school on, few have not been subjected to taunting by white classmates, fingers pulling out the corners of their own eyes to what must be a painful slant. Asian American women, exposed to the visual rhetoric of American beauty magazines, learn quickly that large, deep-set, heavy-lidded eyes are the standard toward which they ought to wield their arsenal of cosmetics. Asian American

women's eyes are the site of images that run the proverbial gamut: slant-eye Jap and sloe-eyed beauty, the mysteriously lidded eye that conceals nefarious intelligence and the weird slit that promises a weirder and titillating slit below.[48]

"Asian eyes"—categorically ingrained as a singular eye shape—assumes racial homogeneity. What fashion magazine aimed at white women has not included at least one obligatory article advising Asian women to use purple eye-shadow to make small eyes look bigger? Though 50 percent of Asian people do "have the fold," the assumption, which Yamamoto critiques, is that all Asian people have the same eye shape. Racism only allows Asian people to see through a lidless eye. Still, statistics on how many Asian people do or don't have the fold are largely irrelevant, since the real problem lies in the racialized move that equates "stereotyped genetic physical features ('small, slanty' eyes and a 'flat' nose) with negative behavioral characteristics."[49]

In April 2000, the *NewsHour with Jim Lehrer* interviewed seven white, male U.S. senators who served in the Vietnam War for *Legacy*, a series of news stories commemorating the twenty-fifth anniversary of the fall of Saigon.[50] The senators, both Democrats and Republicans, answered a series of questions on what they learned from serving in Vietnam and how the experience changed their lives. Bob Kerrey, then senator of Nebraska, stated that his world became larger as he traveled thousands of miles across the ocean to fight for people whose "eye shape was different and were a different color and spoke a different language."

Eye shape takes center stage as a marker of racial difference, and he points that out to signify his increased understanding or cosmopolitanism. Kerrey's remarks reduce national difference to bodily signifiers and reassign "whiteness" to the center. Obviously, he could not just claim that the Vietnamese were people of an identifiable and different color, since descriptions of the "yellowness" and sometimes "brownness" of Asian bodies confuses the familiarity of a black-and-white racial matrix. In order to name the Vietnamese without referring to color as national identity, Kerrey reverted to eye shape as the universal indicator of Vietnamese racial, cultural, and national difference.[51]

The line, "One of these slits here will be Miss Saigon," accompanies a cast of Asian women wearing G-strings and bikini tops. They execute perfectly timed spread-eagle crotch shots, bend over, grind their pelvises against the Marines, and sing "See my bikini / it's just the right size / don't you enjoy how it rides up my thighs? / Look from behind / it'll knock out your eyes. / I'll show you: / my special trophy of war." They more than suggest that the "slits" referred to are situated somewhere else besides the women's faces, and maybe, just maybe, the audience will get to see them. This overtly pornographic reference to their anatomy normalizes racism and sexism as wholesome family entertainment.

The performance itself contradicts Behr's claim that military prostitution consists of slightly sordid but mostly innocent teenage sexual fantasies. There are major gaps in Behr's romanticized descriptions of prostitution and what is actually depicted on the *Miss Saigon* stage. If *Miss Saigon* is *Madama Butterfly* sans racist overtones, how does one account for the slurs scripted into the former? Even if the racist and sexist comments hurled at the women by the Marines are "realistic," it is unbelievable that real women are unaffected by such treatment and do not experience resentment. In the production, the bar-girls, with the exception of Kim, are having a good time; and Gigi, played by the most buxom female actor in the cast, keeps looking for the right man to "save" her.

Both *The Story of "Miss Saigon"* and *The Making of "Miss Saigon"* include extensive accounts by Boublil and Schönberg of the cast's overall enthusiasm for the musical's material, as well as the Filipina cast members' reluctance to perform sexually explicit material. Behr and Steyn attribute this reluctance to their Catholic backgrounds and not to the fact that the material might actually be racially and sexually offensive to Asian women. On the one hand, Boublil and Schönberg claim to understand why young Filipina women would not want to be mistaken for prostitutes, and try to convince the women that no such misunderstanding will take place. In the same breath, they also stress the significance of the lead role, Kim, as an archetype of Asian femininity. In an interesting turn, both *The Story of "Miss Saigon"* and *The Making of "Miss Saigon"* describe the Filipina women in the cast as variations on Kim: innocent young girls who must be cajoled into performing as bargirls. Though reluctant at first, they become adept and eventually learn to enjoy the part, as they become worldly in experience while remaining morally innocent.[52]

An article chronicling Melanie Tojio's rise from an unknown dancer to

Lea Salonga's understudy appeared in *Vogue* magazine in June 1991. "Broadway Baby" begins with the declaration that "because she is Asian, because she is short, and because she is from Hawaii, Melanie Tojio never dreamed she'd be on Broadway."[53] "Race" is the operative word in the first statement, because it clearly identifies Asian-ness as a reason why one would not appear in a Broadway production. There is no mention of any deficiencies in talent or overall physical attractiveness—the two factors used to evaluate the potential starlet, and the lack of which signal automatic exclusion from success as a Broadway star. Tojio's race is articulated as the most "obvious" category for exclusion.

The producers of *Miss Saigon* attempted to bill the show as theater that engaged with larger political issues, including antiwar sentiments, yet tried to separate "artistic" concerns from contemporary politics. Van Meter *structures* the *Vogue* article as a series of diary entries, as told by Tojio, documenting everything from the audition to opening night on Broadway. Tojio even offers her view of the casting controversy:

> "Everybody feels for the Asians in New York, including me. I know how hard it is to get a job when you're an Asian. . . . I think in Hawaii the idea's a little different because there's not so much racial tension here. But I understand what people in New York, the Asian actors guild, are going through. This is a good opportunity for them to make a statement and try to help their cause. But I just hope this isn't going to hurt the production."[54]

This is an odd set of statements, since Tojio acknowledges race as the very category that prevents her from imagining that she could ever have been cast in a Broadway production. Yet, the Asian actors in New York City are cast as subjects experiencing a different kind of racism, while Tojio herself accepts the rationale for her previous exclusion from the Broadway stage.

Does the fact that Tojio, a Japanese American woman, was cast despite racism prove that racism on Broadway no longer exists? Are Asian actors supposed to be grateful that someone has written a musical with a racial quota, a Broadway version of affirmative action for Asian Americans? The musical's plot takes place in Asia, and the producers' interpretation of that setting is that at least 25 percent of the cast would "ideally" be Asian people.

If the musical is about the Vietnam War, and if the characters are written as either Vietnamese or American characters, why are Asians limited to 25 percent of the cast? "Casting, at this stage, was still a long way off. This was a challenge: a quarter of the performers had to look like authentic Vietnamese —and they had to be able to sing a complicated, demanding score."[55]

Dramatizing the discovery of Lea Salonga and a pool of Filipina cohorts, *The Making of "Miss Saigon"* claims an inability to locate adequate Asian singing and acting talent. Given the numerous casts performing in cities all over the world, we now know that the perceived labor shortage has been solved. The role of bar-girl, however, has become a dead-end job: an Asian woman has reached the zenith of a Broadway career if she gets a chance to gyrate in a G-string. Similar to Behr's romanticized account of prostitution, Tojio's interview includes a description of trips to strip joints in New York City as research. She realizes, "It's a degrading job, and you have to think of it as such"; which is a far cry from how much fun she has rehearsing the role of the bar-girl with the men in the cast. Later, Tojio provides an account in which the actor playing Chris is instructed to act trashier toward her. He says: "There she is. Come on, give it to me, you bitch."[56] Tojio reports feeling degraded, even though it was just a rehearsal.

Behr's claim that *Miss Saigon* is an accurate portrayal of Vietnamese prostitution justifies the spectacularization of oppression for the purpose of a doubled sexual commodification. The dancers onstage stop just short of stripping down to complete nudity and, in essence, function as soft-porn striptease for the audience. It is not the fact that the scene is sexual that is shocking, but the way in which the scene, purportedly critical of degradation and exploitation, becomes a toe-tapping number. Rather than witnessing a scene that exposes the women's degradation, the audience is presented with an unproblematized and pleasurable spectacle at the expense of the Asian female actors and the women that they portray.

If Boublil and Shöenberg want the audience to believe in the contemporary plausibility of a late-twentieth-century Madame Butterfly, *Miss Saigon's* women must be working girls and Kim a working single mom. The relationship between prostitution and motherhood in *Miss Saigon* is personalized and embodied by Chris and Kim, and depersonalized through the temporal and spatial disembodiment of photographs. Chris and Kim's love affair is a fictional adaptation of a literary and operatic referent, whereas "real Vietnamese people" appear in a slide show of Amerasian children photographed in Vietnamese orphanages.

The scene is Atlanta in 1978, three years after Chris has left Vietnam during the chaotic fall of Saigon. Since his departure, Kim, who has given birth to their son, is still holding onto the dream that Chris will one day return to Asia and rescue her. In the meantime, Kim and her son survive an escape from Vietnam by boat, and Kim, now in Bangkok, resumes her work as a bar-girl. While working under the auspices of her biracial pimp (The Engineer), John, Chris's former superior officer, learns of her whereabouts. John had originally "purchased" Kim for Chris at the Dreamland. Played by a racially interchangeable character, John has embarked on a postwar repentance project to reunite orphaned Amerasian children with their American fathers.

A huge screen fills the stage; images of three-year-old children flash on the screen one after another. It is interesting to note that, very often, the only Vietnamese person consistently cast in the show plays Tam (Kim and Chris's toddler). John stands facing the audience, delivering his speech in song: "I never thought one day I'd plead for half-breeds from a land that's torn. / But then I saw a camp for children whose crime was being born." At this point, there is not a dry eye in the audience. The intangible ravages of American guilt are dealt with by actors portraying their regret through images of the absent. This is the antiwar narrative: a continual stream of black-and-white photos depicting helpless children. The U.S. soldiers who fathered these children are geographically and temporally no longer part of a military-industrial complex, but simply a group of delinquent fathers who owe lots of child support.

The story of the Vietnamese woman who turns to prostitution out of economic need is not contained within the staged context of performing for U.S. soldiers. Her family's tragedy morphs into family entertainment as she executes her spectacular dance numbers for the audience in the theater. U.S. soldiers are portrayed as individuals who work through their guilt by dealing with the realities and consequences of war through the pseudodocumentary slide show. In contrast, the image of the Vietnamese woman is that of a career prostitute who remains cheerful against all odds. Within the narrative of the musical, she continues to entertain her clients with skill; her performance for her clients eventually becomes indistinguishable from the entertainment quotient of the musical itself. Her dance moves from the strip joint to the theater, spilling onto the audience's lap.

Asian women—represented as always on the verge of casually turning to prostitution, during any time of economic uncertainty—are not entirely sympathetic characters. It is hard to make the connection between wartime prostitution and poverty, exploitation, and oppression when the cast of bargirls reappears in a glitzy dream sequence complete with a Cadillac and Miss Chinatown riding shotgun. This chorus of happy hookers is set off by the one unsure virgin. Kim's marriage-like arrangement with Chris is the fabled goal of Asian prostitution—the thing that Western men need to "watch out" for. She returns to the brothel as a tragic whore when her American "husband" leaves the country without her. It is ultimately the American soldier who can save her from the service that he is paying for.

Miss Saigon dabbles in soft porn, with just the right number of strip-joint dance sequences to offset the tear-jerking antiwar sentiments and the inevitable death of the heroine. She is a chaste prostitute, forever childlike, naïve, and blindly trusting, in spite of her "chosen" occupation. Happily dancing in her G-string for audiences around the world, the image of the teenage prostitute reinforces the notion of war as coincidental backdrop to an effeminized and infantilized Asia serving as low-budget whorehouse to the West. In the libretto, our heroine Kim is just seventeen when she turns her first trick. Babies having babies—this is the stuff of American daytime talk shows: Jenny Jones, Sally Jesse Rafael, Montel Williams. But this particular child prostitute/bride barely registers in a nation otherwise obsessed with televising the crisis of teenage sex and parenthood as spectacle.

Behr writes of teenage prostitution as normal sexual experimentation, typical of adolescents:

> The extreme youth of the GIs in Vietnam has been hammered home in countless books and films about the war. The girls were often even younger: both sides were inexperienced, unprepared for tragedy, full of absurd juvenile buoyancy, and the mercantile aspect of bar-girl sex didn't preclude moments of pure joy.[57]

He implies that it is natural for American GIs to discover their sexuality with a Vietnamese prostitute—just as any regular American teenage boys would want to "do it" with the teenage girls willing to "put out." Asian girls, on the other hand, as Behr would have it, define their sexuality through prostitution and, thus, "the mercantile aspect of bar-girl sex didn't preclude moments of pure joy." The Asian sex-tour and mail-order bride industries feed off of the same set of racist assumptions about the nature of Asian womanhood deployed in *Miss Saigon*. Since Asian womanhood is undifferentiated from girlhood, teenage prostitution is a reasonable enough basis for a love story in which the conditions of Kim's occupation are easily overlooked and viewed as emotionally and economically normative.

Kim is a tragic figure because she is not a completely willing whore, like Gigi or the streetwise and calculating prostitutes in *Cabaret* and *Sweet Charity*. A virgin at heart, Kim's ambivalence takes place in front of a backdrop of real professionals who strut on cue. Kim is the perfect Asian woman—unliberated, naïve, and always one song away from the jiggling flesh that keeps the show from becoming overly depressing. Even when she laments her situation, Chris is her savior from Asian-style patriarchy, a fate worse than prostitution. Imperialist discourse locates the fantasy of sex with white men—and not feminism—as a liberatory ideology. Justifying prostitution justifies colonization in the service of rescuing Asia(n women) from cultural backwardness (Asian men).

Is *Miss Saigon* Asian American?

I think it is fairly evident that Boublil and Schönberg did not create *Miss Saigon* with Asian American politics in mind; however, the musical worms its way into any discussion about Asian Americans and the theater. In the world of theatrical What Ifs, one can wonder whether Kim would have ended up Asian American if her creators had not killed her off. The musical itself poses the opportunity to ponder the possibility of an Asian American Dream. In Act II, after Saigon has fallen into the hands of communists, The Engineer finds himself marginally employed on the streets of Bangkok, where he falls into a dream sequence ("The American Dream") that includes a chorus of Asian showgirls in blonde wigs and G-strings, reprising choreography reminiscent of "The Heat Is On."

The song-and-dance culminates with the appearance of a Cadillac convertible from which a blonde Miss Chinatown, dressed like the Statue of

Liberty, beckons The Engineer to join her in the car. If the writers meant this to be The Engineer's warped vision of a generic America, it is Asian America that experiences the warping. For it is Miss Chinatown, a symbol of diasporic community, acculturation, and ethnic propriety, who provides the lure for the morally depraved, emotionally bankrupt, and desperate Engineer. He is not interested in the ideas associated with such myths of America as freedom, equality, and safety, but with the economic opportunity provided by the body of an Asian American woman sexualized through the eyes of white men. This is *Miss Saigon*'s proposition to Asian America: be grateful for one's good fortune in making it to America. It asks Asian Americans to be complacent, uncomplaining model minorities and to be thankful for a chance to shimmy in the spotlight while projecting gratitude with a smile.

Club O' Noodles's encounter with *Miss Saigon* in *Laughter* works by juxtaposing clear distinctions between fiction and possible reality. If the pedagogy of *Miss Saigon* positions itself as both a history lesson on the Vietnam War and the Western operatic tradition, Club O' Noodles's counterproposal is thematic and choreographic. Its deconstruction of the musical demonstrates the failure of cohesive narratives to account for life stories rife with interruption and memories riddled with gaps.

The fate of works such as *Laughter* remains in question—given the economics of working in an alternative performance milieu—whereas *Miss Saigon* continues its staged existence and its exponential growth. Revisiting *Miss Saigon* helps clarify what is at stake in Club O' Noodles's work as Asian American dancetheater. *Miss Saigon* makes evident the continued presence of the Oriental dancing girl and its affects on the marginalization of Asian and Asian American women, as well as on Asian American artistic subjectivities.

Epilogue

Not one to give *Miss Saigon* the last word, I would like to offer a different ending. I would like to end with an analysis of Maura Nguyen Donohue's *Lotus Blossom Itch* (1997) as an example of choreography that offers a multivalent critique of modern dance history, the trope of the Oriental dancing girl, sex tourism, *Miss Saigon*, anthropology, and the social expectations of community theater. If Sue Li-Jue missed the "Asian American mark," Club O' Noodles missed the "technique mark," and "The Amazing Chinese American Acrobat" waffled between the two as an intellectual exercise, then Donohue's *Lotus Blossom Itch* provides a provocative spectacle for the politically savvy viewer who also appreciates a well-placed *battement*.

At the conclusion of Donohue's *Lotus Blossom Itch*, the members of her group, In Mixed Company, trickle out onstage dressed in street clothes, ready to leave the theater. The dancers walk past three men in sarongs standing under a spotlight in perfect stillness. Without any regard to the three men, who are frozen in mid-gesture blowing kisses to the audience, the rest of the dancers complain about the evening's performance, the size of the theater, the lack of dressing rooms, the conditions of the bathroom, the choreographer, and each other. In a final moment of frustration, one of the women heading for the building exit explodes in a fit of anger, "I don't want to come back and do the show tomorrow. I'm not even getting paid. I'm fuckin' tired of being a lotus blossom pussy!"

This final choreographed outburst near the end of Donohue's forty-minute critique of the trope of the Orientalized dancing girl embodies the encounter between Asian Americans and dance history. It gestures toward performance and choreography as forms of representation as well as representational practices. The men frozen in time are still "in the performance," while the dancers perform the post-performance kvetch. The staging of these two different temporal moments signals the aesthetic boundaries that the work draws upon: performance art, modern dance, and theater. The dancer who is "sick and tired of being the lotus blossom pussy" refuses to be the silent dancing body, even though she has just spent the evening playing the role. This paradox speaks to the way in which the lotus blossom image is a site for critique because it reflects how Asian American bodies performing onstage are caught in a web of representational histories. The lotus blossom provides the backdrop for Asian American dancetheater's potential for subverting dominant histories of U.S. modern dance, and for its limits.

Lotus Blossom Itch performs the invisibilized Orientalism of early-twentieth-century U.S. modern dance and its colonial origins in the guise of human exhibits. Like St. Denis, who merged highbrow appropriations of Eastern spirituality with lowbrow vaudeville dance routine, Donohue borrows a similar tactic, albeit with differing results. Choreographically, Donohue uses "exotic dancing" as a point of reference to investigate the ways in which exotic subjects are perceived as foreign, sensuous, and sexually available. She investigates how "world, ethnic, folk, or cultural" dance forms are used as shortcuts indicating expressions of ethnic identity as well as stereotypes of ethnic identity.

Donohue's most provocative use of choreography illuminates the similarities between the package-tour industry's marketing of world dance forms as signifiers of essentialized ethnic-as-national identity and those of the sex-tour industry's marketing of racially essentialized pornography. Choreographically, Donohue asks, "What makes an Oriental massage Oriental?" Donohue offers an array of Oriental dancing girls—hula dancers in grass skirts and coconut shells, natives in natural habitats doing mating dances, and Salome and her seven veils—to demonstrate the range with which the dancing Asian body has been imagined in the service of sexual fantasy. For Donohue, these sexualized bodies are ultimately informed by discourses of militarized prostitution. At work in *Lotus Blossom Itch* is the ever-present specter of *Miss Saigon*—the blockbuster Broadway musical that continues to entertain the world with its recycled Madame Butterfly narrative sung by a cast of scantily clad Filipino women playing Vietnamese bar-girls.

Lotus Blossom Itch begins with a greeting by three Asian American men wearing sarongs. Two of them drum on guitars as they welcome and inform the audience that they are about to embark on a scheduled departure of Fantasy Tour B. The audience is taken on a "tour" of exotic Asian cultures through the lenses of sexual voyeurism, cultural appropriation, and consumerism. Donohue unearths the intertwined history between Orientalism in high-art Western dance vocabularies and the trope of the exotic, erotic, Oriental dancing girl. The three men act as tour guides, explaining to the audience that Fantasy Tour B is an all-inclusive vacation package and the first stop is Hawaii. The guides introduce Miss Hawaii and disclose that she is really from St. Louis (pronounced "St. Louie"). Miss Hawaii enters the stage wearing a grass skirt and a bikini top made out of coconut shells. She is flanked by two men wearing loincloths and begins to undulate her arms while gyrating her hips in a mock hula. Donohue combines signifying gestures of hula, modern dance, contact improvisation, and striptease to critique the way in which the "Oriental dancing girl" is easily seen within the framework of a sexual fantasy.

Actual hula vocabulary is interrupted by stereotypical hula movements in order to disrupt a romanticized reading of cross-cultural moments. Since the appropriation of Asian aesthetics is critically invisible within the narrative of a unified American cultural identity, Asian American artistic production is continually read as an attempt to reconcile a conflicted cultural identity between East and West. Asian-ness is always held in diametrical opposition to Western-ness, specifically movement vocabulary and choreographic approaches, despite a century of cultural appropriation. Donohue's choreography critiques the way in which the desire for seeing authentic bodies performing authentic culture is also part of an Orientalist fantasy that easily substitutes costumes for actual people and cultural understanding. Donohue presents a series of cabaret-style "tourist dances" such as the hula, belly dance, and fan dance in order to examine the ways in which the sex-tour and porn industries use Orientalist cultural signifiers to market Orientalized female bodies as a special brand of sexual pleasure.

Miss Hawaii continues her slow-paced undulations while two male dancers beginning stomping and hooting. A voiceover calls attention to the "natives'" authentically dancing in a "primitive" manner, while the two men thrust their hunched torsos back and forth. Movements reminiscent of the perfunctory tourist dance show are now framed by a zoolike context suggestive of the late-nineteenth-century and early-twentieth-century world expositions and the practice of displaying non-white people in fake authentic settings. A voiceover announces that souvenirs can be purchased in the gift shop after the tour. One of the men gradually moves the undulations of his torso down his body until he is executing a series of pelvic thrusts. He starts dancing as if he is stripping, while the other man maintains his primitive dancing. Eventually the man thrusting his pelvis back and forth ends up standing near or behind Miss Hawaii. The men alternate between primitive dancing and erotic dancing as a comment on a history of anthropological studies and the construction of racial otherness. The scene is also reminiscent of ethnographic films that attempt to document "native life." These films often frame non-Western people in the same way that wildlife documentaries frame their subjects: they focus on how people hunt for food, sleep, eat, get dressed, and ultimately reproduce.

Choreographically, Donohue uses both high-art and low-art dance vocabularies to reveal the close connections among the tourist dance-show, the sex-tour industry, striptease, modern dance, and contact improvisation. She references the legacies of early modern dancers, such as Isadora Duncan and particularly Ruth St. Denis. Donohue's choreography is a critique of an American modern and postmodern dance history that—under the guise of depoliticization, "artistic innovation," and "abstraction"—has rendered invisible its continual cycle of Orientalism. Donohue exposes the way in which movement vocabularies—such as contact improvisation, with its reputation for democracy, being in the moment, experiencing movement, and access to an intellectually and spiritually enlightened alternative lifestyle—masks Orientalist appropriations that have marked every significant shift in American dance history. We recall Ruth St. Denis's pan-Orientalist dances, Martha Graham's fascination with Asian female dancing bodies, Merce Cunningham and the *I Ching,* Judson Church's claims to Zen-like mindsets, and contact improvisation's foundation of aikido. The historical trajectory of high-art American dance idioms depends upon an impulse to create choreography for a sophisticated audience who can intellectually appreciate movement vocabulary without the baggage of mainstream social contexts. Donohue choreographs against the move toward abstraction.

Ruth St. Denis's interpretations of the Orient provided American modern dance with an opportunity for artistic legitimacy. Her pursuits did not occur in an artistic vacuum. Instead, her choreography is part of the political continuum in which the fantasy of interracial sex involving geishas and other renditions of Asian female prostitutes retains its popular appeal. These images fuel a booming market for sex tours in Asia and Hawaii, the mail-order bride industry, and sanctioned military prostitution. Asian prostitution is racially differentiated from prostitution in general, such that young Asian women and girls are considered to have an unproblematic affinity for sex work.

Later in *Lotus Blossom Itch*, we are presented with Salome and her seven veils. A woman wearing a gold lamé bikini top and a skirt made out of scarves comes out on stage. She begins removing her veils one by one. She gestures at Middle Eastern dancing while drawing attention to her scantily clad body. She takes the scarves off of her skirt and runs them over her body before throwing them into the air. Other scantily clad female dancers run onstage trailing scarves behind them and a voiceover announces "Isadora," just as Salome turns her back to the audience and kicks up her leg while reaching toward the sky with her arms. Moments later, the voiceover announces "Ruth St. Denis" and "Denishawn" when a male dancer in harem pants enters to dance with Salome. The lights dim and, instead of continuing to remove her veils one by one, Salome places a hand on her waist and forcefully rips off her entire skirt, exposing her gold lamé G-string. While Salome has her back to the audience, the voiceover announces that it is real, 100 percent gold lamé and can be purchased in the gift shop.

Salome and her partner execute a duet while rolling on the floor and lifting each other. Behind them is a larger group, dimly lit, crawling and sliding over one another in a slow, oozing mass. Salome has abandoned her Oriental movement vocabulary and both groups are leaning on, pushing, falling, and rolling over one another, as in contact improvisation. The costumes (or lack thereof) and music draw attention to the dancers' compromising positions. The choreography uses contact improvisation's sex-like dance vocabulary to call attention to the sexualized imagery informing the development of American modern and postmodern dance. The scene becomes essentially a live sex show featuring both a heterosexual couple and a group orgy, while the voiceover continues to remind spectators that souvenirs can be purchased in the gift shop. The sexual innuendo in these constant verbal reminders points to the way in which the success of the sex-tour industry depends on the rationalization of sexual exploitation as a necessary component of global capitalism. Donohue mirrors this rationalization in her evocation of Oriental dance, cabaret-style belly dance, contact improvisation, and the sex act. Choreographically, Donohue makes use of different movement vocabularies to demonstrate the similar ways that exoticism functions in the seemingly different contexts of highbrow concert dance and the seedy strip club.

One of the tour's stops is "China"; it features a real-life China Doll wearing the top half of a silky red pajama suit—the kind found in Chinatown tourist gift shops. The dancer holds a large fan reminiscent of Linda Low's "Fan-tan Fanny" number from *Flower Drum Song,* or a stereotypical burlesque act involving large, feathered fans held strategically to hide a dancer's implied nude torso. The voiceover announces in a matter-of-fact tone that "red is the color of love in China," as the dancer opens and closes her fan. She then slides her legs into second-position splits (a move that is often referred to by its more popular terminology, the "Chinese splits"), and crawls on the ground. Red, a color associated with weddings in China, with communism, and with Asia in general, is sexualized using an American reference to Valentine's Day and the commodification of sex and romance. The movement of the dancer's legs sliding into the splits gestures to ways in which random Asian cultural signifiers (in this case, the color red) and stereotypes (the association of extreme flexibility with Chinese-ness) can be easily nuanced with sexual overtones in the sex industry. It is a way of marketing a kind of racist multicultural porn.

In the finale, Donohue herself appears on stage, but this time the scene is not an exotic Asian locale but a strip joint in New York City's Times Square. Dressed in a black top and a conical straw hat, she performs the role of a stripper who is performing as a Vietnamese prostitute dressed like a peasant. It is an actual strip act in the sense that she ends up topless at the conclusion of her solo. The choreography is based on Donohue's research working in a strip joint. She uses a few props to create her stage persona, because racialized imagery of wartime prostitution can now be worn as a costume. The rest of the company members come out on stage dressed in skimpy latex dresses or shorts, executing Broadway-style choreography in unison. It is hard not to interpret this last section of the choreography as a reference to *Miss Saigon*'s status as legitimate theater, popular culture, tourist attraction, and Asian employment opportunity.

Donohue reappropriates St. Denis's Orientalism to make a choreographic critique of the way in which cultural appropriation makes it difficult to see dancing Asian female bodies outside of the parameters of the "Oriental dancing girl." Even in executing a supposedly abstract movement vocabulary, Donohue exposes the mechanisms through which the Asian female body is easily put back into the frame of Orientalism. She also critiques the way the sex industry racializes Asian female bodies via narratives of culturally inflected sexual exoticism. Donohue's criticisms are overt and the work is politically and sexually explicit. She pairs model-minority cultural behavior in the form of "traditional" dances with professionalized sex, while the model-minority-as-economic powerhouse lurks in her critique of global capitalism and Asian female labor.

In staging the encounter between modern dance history and Asian American critique, *Lotus Blossom Itch* creates space for questioning the choreographic conventions deployed in the dance itself. Just as the ending calls attention to the staged nature of the performance event, the critique of St. Denis, Shawn, and Duncan questions the notion of movement invention. If each subsequent generation of modern-dance choreographers has "broken away" from its dance training, it has always been done with the belief that something new could be developed, accessed, discovered, retrieved, or adapted. One worked with the faith that something new would follow, be it "authentic," as in the Authentic Movement, or entirely contrived, as in digitized computer programs. Donohue opens the door to thinking about the distance between dancing and Asian American critique.

To write about Asian American dance is to work at the intersection between two discourses. One history sees itself as a lineage of form, while the other sees itself as a politics of representation. It is true that form may, in fact, be political, but to the practitioners of form this may not matter. Similarly, the proponents of the political may be more concerned with the repercussions of representation than with form. Writing about Asian American dance involves negotiating two fields that do not register with each other, such that an Asian American critique of dance history is like holding two simultaneous but separate conversations. I am reminded of Trisha Brown's *Talking Plus Watermotor,* in which Brown alternates between telling two stories while executing two movement phrases. There is only one body performing both narratives and phrases, but the narratives and the phrases remain unaffected by one another. What the audience sees is Brown's phenomenal skill in keeping track. Her body does the work of showing the work, but the individual stories and phrases she performs retain their own identities even in the presence of one another.

What I have attempted to indicate in this book is the scope of "performing research," which includes the intellectual work of engaging disciplinary audiences who are not typically in conversation with one another. Performing research also involves getting caught up in the creative process as an important component in the analysis of representation. The tension between fixing performed representation into an object of textual analysis and the belief in the ongoing-ness of performance is at the crux of Asian American dance studies. The discourse of dance is centered around literal and figurative mobility—where something cannot be fixed or thoroughly explained. To do so would ruin what pleasure dancing can offer in its ephemerality and thus nonspecificity. Without a tangible identity, dance, then, is slippery and elusive. It asserts the ability to be anything and everything, existing outside of the banality of politics, social norms, and history.

The history of modern dance—in its claim to the modern, the here, and the presence of the dancing body—is essentially a story about erasing the past. As a discourse, Asian American studies takes up the opposite view of performance; ultimately, it is all about representation. Asian American dance artists offer an alternative view of performance by working within the open conceptual framework of contemporary dance. Their work has the potential to generate layers of meaning, to take on both the presence of the body and issues of representation—thereby challenging previously durable stereotypes and taking us to a deeper understanding of Asian America.

NOTES

Introduction

1. See Renny Christopher, *The Viet Nam War/The American War: Images and Representations in Euro-American and Vietnamese Exile Narratives* (Amherst: University of Massachusetts Press, 1995); and Michael Anderegg, ed., *Inventing Vietnam: The War in Film and Television* (Philadelphia: Temple University Press, 1991). Both authors discuss the way in which the American public's unfamiliarity with the complex politics of the Vietnam War, coupled with Hollywood representations of the war, manipulated the public's desire to conflate all Vietnamese people with the enemy North Vietnamese army. The arrival of Vietnamese refugees and immigrants after the fall of Saigon in 1975 posed an ideological problem for an American public hostile to Asian immigration, particularly that of Asians recently depicted as "the enemy."

2. Josephine Lee, *Performing Asian America: Race and Ethnicity on the Contemporary Stage* (Philadelphia: Temple University Press, 1997), 24.

3. It is true that the bulk of publications in these fields are biographical. Within the field of Asian American studies, there is a lack of biographical writings about writers and artists in general. Biographical studies in dance tend to identify individual artists and their artistic legacies. Asian American literary studies challenges modernist notions of artistic achievement. Josephine Lee follows this literary approach and resists the reinscription of an Asian American theater canon by refusing to engage in a discussion of the artistic merits of individual plays. She writes, "I purposefully avoid any attempts to create an alternative canon, to rank the individual masterpiece, or to assess the excellence of any writer." She does this to avoid placing on any one piece the "burden of representation," in which individual Asian American writers are held responsible to represent the entirety of the Asian American experience. See Josephine Lee, *Performing Asian America,* 6–7.

4. Ping Chong and Muna Tseng, "SlutForArt," in *Tokens? The NYC Asian American Experience on Stage*, ed. Alvin Eng (New York: Asian American Writers Workshop, 1999), 378–405.

5. Maura Donohue, "When You're Old Enough," in *Watermark: Vietnamese American Poetry and Prose*, ed. Barbara Tran, Monique T. D. Truong, and Luu Truong Khoi (New York: Asian American Writers Workshop, 1998), 108.

6. Chong and Tseng, "SlutForArt," 384.

7. Susan Foster, "Choreographing History: A Manifesto for Dead and Moving

Bodies," in *Choreographing History,* ed. Susan Foster (Bloomington: Indiana University Press, 1995), 3.

8. Dorinne Kondo, *About Face: Performing Race in Fashion and Theater* (New York: Routledge, 1997), 20.

9. Johannes Fabian, *Power and Performance: Ethnographic Explorations through Proverbial Wisdom and Theater in Shaba, Zäire* (Madison: University of Wisconsin Press, 1990), 11.

10. Richard Dyer, "The Role of Stereotypes," in *The Matter of Images: Essays on Representations* (New York: Routledge, 1993), 1.

11. See Christopher, *The Viet Nam War;* Anderegg, *Inventing Vietnam;* and n. 1.

12. See Lisa Lowe, *Immigrant Acts: On Asian American Cultural Politics* (Durham, N.C.: Duke University Press, 1996), for a complete discussion of anti-Asian immigration legislation and the formation of the Asian American subject as a perpetual foreigner.

13. Ibid., 91.

14. See Martin Manalansan IV's critique of fusion cuisine as the new Orientalism and the ways in which Asian Americans are racialized through discourses of containment and consumption of "ethnic food": "Cooking up the Senses: A Critical Embodied Approach to the Study of Food and Asian American Television Audiences," in *Alien Encounters: Popular Culture in America,* ed. Mimi Thi Nguyen and Thuy Linh Nguyen Tu (Durham, N.C.: Duke University Press, 2007): 179–93.

15. Johannes Fabian, "Presence and Representation (1990)," in *Time and the Work of Anthropology: Critical Essays 1971–1991* (Chur, Switzerland: Harwood Academic Publishers, 1991), 207.

16. Ibid., 209.

17. Ibid.

18. Edward Said, *Orientalism* (New York: Vintage Books, 1979), 233.

19. James S. Moy, *Marginal Sights: Staging the Chinese in America* (Iowa City: University of Iowa Press, 1993), 39.

20. Said, *Orientalism,* 6.

21. See Sarah Strauss, *Positioning Yoga: Balancing Acts Across Culture* (Oxford: Berg Publishers, 2005), for a history of yoga's introduction to the West and an analysis of yoga as a global industry.

22. The internment of Japanese Americans during World War II is a case in point, as is the racial profiling of Muslims and Arab Americans after September 11, 2001.

23. See Sucheta Mazumdar, "General Introduction: A Woman-Centered Perspective on Asian American History," in *Making Waves: An Anthology of Writings by and about Asian American Women,* ed. Asian Women United of California (Boston: Beacon Press, 1989), 13; Deborah Woo, "The Gap Between Striving and Achieving: The Case of Asian American Women," in Asian Women United, *Making Waves,* 185–94.

24. Jun Xing, *Asian America Through the Lens: Representations, History, and Identity* (Walnut Creek, Calif.: Altamira Press, 1998), 14.

25. Robert G. Lee, *Orientals: Asian Americans in Popular Culture* (Philadelphia: Temple University Press, 1999), 150.

26. Yuko Kurahashi, *Asian American Culture on Stage: The History of the East West Players* (New York: Garland, 1999), 9.

27. R. Lee, *Orientals*, 182–83.

28. Ibid., 175–76.

1. Situating Asian American Dance Studies

1. Personal interview with choreographer, November 2000.

2. Sima Belmar, "Boxed In: *The Nature of Nature* Is Trapped in Stereotypes," *San Francisco Bay Guardian* 35, no. 25 (March 21–27, 2001): 49.

3. Marta E. Savigliano, *Tango and the Political Economy of Passion* (Boulder, Colo.: Westview Press, 1995).

4. Esther Kim Lee, *A History of Asian American Theatre* (Cambridge: Cambridge University Press, 2006), 6.

5. For a comprehensive history of the East West Players, see Yuko Kurahashi's *Asian American Culture on Stage: The History of the East West Players* (New York: Garland, 1999). For a history on the founding of the first four Asian American theater companies, see Esther Kim Lee, "The First Four Theatre Companies," in *A History of Asian American Theatre,* 42–91.

6. For a discussion of the ways in which Indian dance is positioned between discourses of Indian nationalism and modernism, see Ananya Chatterjea, "Danced Disruptions: Postmodern Preoccupations and Reconsiderations," in *Butting Out: Reading the Resistive Choreographies Through Works by Jawole Willa Jo Zollar and Chandralekha.* (Middletown, Conn.: Wesleyan University Press, 2004): 98–134.

7. Shannon Jackson, "Culture and Performance," in *Professing Performance: Theatre in the Academy from Philology to Performativity* (Cambridge: Cambridge University Press, 2004), 83.

8. The direction of dance studies in the 1990s, as represented by collections such as Susan Foster's *Corporealities: Dancing Knowledge, Culture and Power* (New York: Routledge, 1996) and *Choreographing History*, created a dilemma in the field regarding the question of who such works were written for if professional dancers or dance students in pre-professional programs found the work unintelligible.

9. How else can one explain the phenomenon of the claim that an Asian or Asian American actor "must" pay one's dues by acting in roles that reinforce Asian stereotypes?

10. Josephine Lee, *Performing Asian America: Race and Ethnicity on the Contemporary Stage* (Philadelphia: Temple University Press, 1997), 23.

11. Dance scholars Susan Foster and Sally Banes have written about the sexualization of female ballet dancers and the effeminization of male ballet dancers.

12. *Philadelphia Metro,* nos. 16–18 (November 2001): 15. *The Philadelphia Metro* is a free newspaper distributed in Philadelphia's centrally located commuter train terminals. Covering primarily local events and issues, the publication also includes national and international headlines. The photo of Tea appeared inside the paper on the front page of the advertising supplement. The advertising supplement, framed as a holiday guide, provides information about local events such as Santa Claus appearances and places to go Christmas shopping.

13. For a discussion of the way in which choreographers and dancers are representative agents, see Susan Foster's *Choreographing History* and *Reading Dancing* (Berkeley: University of California Press, 1986).

14. Edward Said, *Orientalism* (New York: Vintage Books, 1979), 2–3.

15. Amy Koritz, "Dancing the Orient for England: Maud Allan's 'The Vision of Salome,'" *Theatre Journal* 46, no. 1 (1994): 73.

16. See Gaylyn Studlar, "Out-Salomeing Salome: Dance, the New Woman, and Fan Magazine Orientalism," in *Visions of the East: Orientalism in Film,* ed. Matthew Bernstein and Gaylyn Studlar (New Brunswick, N.J.: Rutgers University Press, 1997), 99–129; and Adrienne L. McLean, "The Thousand Ways There Are to Move," in Bernstein and Studlar, *Visions of the East,* 130–57. Studlar extends Jane Desmond's analysis of St. Denis's Orientalism and investigates the impact of the "Denishawn look" on popular culture. McLean examines Jack Cole's use of camp discourse and Orientalist dance practices to develop a signature style in his 1940s and '50s choreography for Hollywood film.

17. See Walter Terry, *Miss Ruth: The More Living Life of Ruth St. Denis* (New York: Dodd, Mead & Co., 1969), 39–42; Elizabeth Kendall, *Where She Danced* (New York: Alfred A. Knopf, 1979), 34–52; Suzanne Shelton, *Divine Dancer: A Biography of Ruth St. Denis* (Garden City, N.Y.: Doubleday, 1981), 30; Jane Desmond, "Dancing Out the Difference: Cultural Imperialism and Ruth St. Denis' 'Radha' of 1906," *Signs* 17, no. 1 (1991): 28; and Sally Banes, *Dancing Women: Female Bodies on Stage* (New York: Routledge, 1998), 80–92.

18. Banes, *Dancing Women,* 91.

19. Ronald Takaki, *Strangers from a Different Shore: A History of Asian Americans* (New York: Penguin Books, 1990). Takaki's classic text outlines the history of anti-Asian immigration laws.

20. Chinese men were accused of a genetic propensity for homosexuality because the Chinese population in the United States was predominantly male and did not form nuclear families. Accusers ignored the fact that U.S. immigration laws barred Chinese women from entering the United States, and antimiscegenation laws forbade interracial marriage.

21. Shelton, *Divine Dancer*, 95–96.

22. In 1852, there were seven Chinese men to every Chinese female in California. Two decades later, the ratio of Chinese men to women increased to fourteen to one. In 1870, 61 percent of Chinese women in the United States were prostitutes, the majority of whom were forced into the sex trade as indentured servants in order to pay off debts for their passage from China to the United States. By 1880, the number of Chinese prostitutes in California reported in census documents fell to 24 percent of the total Chinese female population. Prostitutes were oftentimes unable to pay off their debts since their terms of service could be extended indefinitely in the event of inevitable illnesses and/or pregnancies. The women were susceptible to venereal diseases and many died from physical abuse, drug overdose, or suicide. See Takaki, *Strangers,* 120–23.

23. I would include the current "war on terror" to the list of race wars. In her essay on performances of Arab-face by American belly dancers in San Francisco, Sunaina Maira observes that the increased popularity of Middle Eastern belly dance and the various practices of fusion forms do not necessarily translate into increased knowledge or awareness of contemporary Middle Eastern culture or politics. Instead many practitioners of belly dance subscribe to Orientalist perceptions of the Middle East as uniformly despotic, oppressive, and backwards. Quite often, American women claim to adopt belly dance as a way to access an alluring yet safe sensuality (Middle Eastern femininity). Much like St. Denis's performance of *nautch* girls and other Oriental dance girl personas performed for white, middle-class audiences, sensuality is made safe by removing oneself from the dangerous sexuality posed by Middle Eastern men. For a full discussion see Sunaina Maira, "Belly Dancing: Arab-Face, Orientalist Feminism and U.S. Empire," *American Quarterly* 60, no. 2 (June 2008): 317–45.

24. Doris Hering, review of the Asian New Dance Coalition, Sun Ock Lee's Studio, *Dance Magazine* (July 1979): 106–8.

25. Bill Moore, "Asian Balm," *Other Stages* (April 1983), n.p.

26. Margaret O'Keefe, "Asian American Dance Theatre," *Attitude: The Dancer's Monthly* 2, no. 1 (June 1983): 10.

27. Rosemary Newton, "Choreographer of the Month: Saeko Ichinohe," *Attitude: The Dancer's Monthly* 2, no. 3 (August 1983): 10.

2. Club O' Noodles's *Laughter from the Children of War*

1. Lisa Lowe, *Immigrant Acts: On Asian American Cultural Politics* (Durham, N.C.: Duke University Press, 1996), 84–96.

2. Clifford Geertz, "Thick Description: Toward an Interpretive Theory of Culture," in *The Interpretation of Cultures: Selected Essays* (New York: Basic Books, 1973), 330. I am extending Geertz's discussion of thick description to account for the reading

of choreography (Susan L. Foster, *Reading Dancing* [Berkeley: University of California Press, 1986]) as an ethnographic encounter. Geertz's analysis of Gilbert Ryle's discussion about the difference between a twitch and a wink poses a similar set of questions when applied to multigenre performance. Given the focus on text-based analyses of performance in Asian American studies, I employ thick description of stage direction and choreography in order to call attention to textual analysis as a form of ethnographic interpretation.

3. Dance scholar Sally Banes has argued that the "postmodern" in "postmodern dance" corresponds with modernist aesthetic concerns in other art forms, such as painting. See *Terpsichore in Sneakers,* 2nd ed. (Middletown, Conn.: Wesleyan University Press, 1987).

4. During rehearsals, the performers would talk about whether or not a character seemed "real" in reference to themselves or someone they knew. In one instance, the director told a woman that she was overdoing it, to which the actor responded, "That's really what my mother sounds like."

5. During rehearsals, the performers would discuss which scenes or combination of scenes determined the content of *Laughter.*

6. *Laughter from the Children of War*, dir. Hung Nguyen and Nobuko Miyamoto, University of California–Riverside, videotape, 16 May 1996. Unless otherwise indicated, all future references to the performance of this work are cited from this performance.

7. "F.O.B.," or "fresh off the boat," is a derogatory term that designates Asian immigrants who are not "Americanized." It is usually used to characterize individuals and groups of recent immigrants with limited English skills, who speak with a heavy Asian accent or who display social behaviors that are characterized as un-American. The term also implies lack of sophistication in regard to familiarity with "normative" American culture. "Fresh off the boat" refers to un-Americanized behavior by any immigrant; but in the case of Vietnamese refugees, the term is ironic because, in fact, many of them escaped Vietnam by boat. Thus, when applied to Vietnamese immigrants, "F.O.B." becomes literal. In addition, it signals class and regional differences within the community, given that some came to America by plane because of their political or social connections.

8. At the end of Renee Tajima-Pena's film *My America, or Honk if You Love Buddha* (1997), she asks the rhetorical question, "What do Asians in America have in common except eating rice?" The 2003–2004 performance project that toured the United States and Asia featuring artists involved with Asia Pacific Performance Exchange (APPEX) was called "The Art of Rice." Focusing on rice as a universal symbol of Asian-ness is obviously a flawed perspective, given the diversity of dietary habits found across different regions and populations.

9. In the following chapters, I will further formulate the concept of "identity" as a

lived experience that is inextricably connected to ideological structures of power. Club O' Noodles struggles to maintain a cohesive group based on an understanding of "Vietnamese American-ness" as a lived reality. This reality is constantly bombarded with information and occurrences that seek simultaneously to reinforce and dismantle the conditions for defining the concept of identity.

10. T. Minh-ha Trinh, *Woman, Native, Other: Writing Postcoloniality and Feminism* (Bloomington: Indiana University Press, 1989), 89.

11. I am using the term "we" to indicate that I was part of the audience present at the performance. My use of "we" is an experiment in imagining different interpretations that could be generated from different subject positions with immigrant communities. My analysis is also based on comments made during the question-and-answer session at the end of the performance and on informal interviews with audience members. I will not undertake an in-depth analysis of the composition of the audience in this book.

12. In 2004, another Hung, William Hung, became both the star and the laughing stock of *American Idol* for his off-key rendition of Ricky Martin's "She Bangs." His public persona as a nerdy, unattractive, tone-deaf, and uncoordinated engineering student at UC Berkeley registers identically with Hollywood stereotypes of Asian men (such as the infamous Long Duk Dong in *Sixteen Candles*). But, in the case of William Hung, his public persona is not an act. Even though seeing failed *American Idol* auditions is part of the program's appeal, why does Hung's failure stand out? One's pleasure in watching footage of *American Idol* rejects is usually understood as the enjoyment of watching a person who suffers from delusions of grandeur and the ensuing argument that the person has with Simon Cowell. William Hung, however, does not argue with Cowell, but concedes that he (Hung) is, in fact, a bad singer. Hung functions as a pathetic character who deserves sympathy when Simon berates him. In this case, Simon's criticisms are not discriminatory (as in telling women they need to lose weight), but Simon has crossed a line because Hung never had a chance. The sympathy Hung manages to generate is similar to that which an audience would feel if Simon made fun of someone developmentally disabled. Such behavior would be out of bounds in terms of good taste; and Hung's condition—nerdy Asian guy—must be treated differently. Hung "trying his best" is infantilized, rendered cute and endearing. His performance provides an opportunity to indulge in the enjoyment of laughing at a racist stereotype without any political backlash because it is, in fact, real.

13. Here I am using the term "choreographic choices" metaphorically to describe Hung Nguyen's verbal performance of accents in a positive manner, in order to bring attention to the fact that "accents" are not the problem, but, rather, the judgment that is passed on the speaker who has an accent.

14. Trinh, *Woman, Native, Other*, 86.

15. For a discussion of the history of cross-racial casting and the complex debates

over color-blind casting practices in theater, see Angela C. Pao, "Changing Faces: Recasting National Identity in All-Asian(-)American Dramas," *Theatre Journal* 53, no. 3 (2001): 389–409.

16. Hung Nguyen, et al., *Laughter from the Children of War*, manuscript, 1997, n.p. All subsequent dialogue in this essay is cited from this script.

17. The title of 2 Live Crew's 1989 album is *As Nasty as They Want to Be.*

18. "White Guy" refers to the character in the play; "White guy" refers to the actor that is needed to play White Guy.

19. See Richard Dyer's discussion of Tarzan and the construction of White masculinity in *The Matter of Images: Essays on Representation* (London: Routledge, 1993).

20. *Laughter* uses excerpts from Andrew Lam's "Love, Money, Prison, Sin, Revenge," *Los Angeles Times Magazine* (March 13, 1994): 24.

21. Ibid.

22. Ibid., 30.

23. Ibid., 26.

24. Trịnh Công Sơn was a celebrated singer/songwriter in Vietnam. Since his death in 2001, his love songs and anti-war songs have remained popular. For an in-depth discussion of the anti-war themes in Trịnh Công Sơn's music see John C. Schafer, "The Trịnh Công Sơn Phenomenon," *Journal of Asian Studies* 66, no. 3 (August 2007): 597–643. Richard Fuller's English translation of "Gia tài của mẹ" can be found at http://www.tcs-home.org/songs-en/songs/a-mother-s-heritage. Accessed 22 April 2009.

25. See Karen Shimakawa's analysis of Ping Chong's *Deshima,* in *National Abjection* (Durham, N.C.: Duke University Press, 2002).

3. Rehearsing the Collective: A Performative Autoethnography

1. Dan Bacalzo, "Collective Autobiographies: The Process of Peeling," paper presented at the Association for Asian American Studies Conference, 31 March 2001, Toronto, Ontario.

2. Johannes Fabian, *Power and Performance: Ethnographic Explorations through Proverbial Wisdom and Theater in Shaba, Zaïre* (Madison: University of Wisconsin Press, 1990).

3. José Esteban Muñoz, "Feeling Brown: Ethnicity and Affect in Ricardo Bràcho's *The Sweetest Hangover (and Other STDs),*" *Theatre Journal: Latino Performance* 52, no. 1 (March 2000): 70.

4. See David Eng, "In the Shadows of the Diva: Committing Homosexuality in David Henry Hwang's *M. Butterfly,*" *Amerasia,* 20, no.1 (1994): 93–116; Dorinne Kondo, "*M. Butterfly*: Orientalism, Gender, and a Critique of Essentialist Identity," *Cultural Critique* 16 (Autumn 1990): 5–29; James S. Moy, "David Henry Hwang's *M.*

Butterfly and Philip Kan Gotanda's *Yankee Dawg You Die*: Repositioning Chinese American Marginality on the American Stage," *Theatre Journal* 42, no. 1 (1990): 48–56; and Josephine Lee, *Performing Asian America: Race and Ethnicity on the Contemporary Stage* (Philadelphia: Temple University Press, 1997), 105–20.

5. Yutian Wong, "Discussion," in *Maps of City and Body*, ed. Denise Uyehara (New York: Kaya Press, 2003), 153–63; and Y. Wong. "Towards a New Asian American Dance Theory," *Discourses in Dance* 1, no. 1 (2002): 69–89.

6. Muñoz characterizes Latino/a affectations of cultural excess as a form of disidentification with normative cultural behavior (Whiteness). The use of excess in the reappropriation and deployment of Latino/a stereotypes decenters Whiteness such that Whiteness represents lack.

7. See D. Eng, "In the Shadows of the Diva"; Kondo, "*M. Butterfly*"; Moy, "David Henry Hwang's *M. Butterfly*"; and Karen Shimakawa, " 'Who's To Say?' or, Making Space for Gender and Ethnicity in *M. Butterfly*," *Theatre Journal* 45, no. 3 (1993): 349–62.

8. "Anh" is a pseudonym. For the purposes of privacy, I use pseudonyms when relating anecdotes that involve the disclosure of personal information. In anecdotes that do not contain personal disclosures, I will use people's first names. For example, in the previous anecdote recounting the choreography of the fight scene, I chose to use people's names since their identities are accessible to the public via program notes, press releases, and the performance itself.

9. See chapter 6, "Pedagogy of the Scantily Clad: Studying *Miss Saigon* in the Twenty-first Century," for an in-depth discussion.

Interlude: *The Amazing Chinese American Acrobat:* Choreography as Methodology

1. James S. Moy, *Marginal Sights: Staging the Chinese in America* (Iowa City: University of Iowa Press, 1993), 130–41.

2. The politics of articulating ethnic identity via national "origins" versus the monolithic term "Asian American" as a political identity is a contentious topic. See Kamala Visweswaran, "Identifying Ethnography," in *Fictions of Feminist Ethnography* (Minneapolis: University of Minnesota Press, 1994).

3. I use Moy because of the passion with which he objects to the Chinese acrobats. The fervor of his objection indicates the degree of investment the writer brings to his spectatorship. Although his concern with authenticity might appear out of fashion in recent Asian American cultural criticism, Moy's focus on this issue speaks to the interests of a general Asian American viewing public.

4. See David L. Eng, "In the Shadows of the Diva: Commiting Homosexuality in David Henry Hwang's *M. Butterfly*," *Amerasia Journal* 20, no. 1 (1994), 93–116; Dar-

rell Y. Hamamoto, *Monitored Peril: Asian Americans and the Politics of TV Representation* (Minneapolis: University of Minnesota Press, 1994); Dorinne K. Kondo, "*M. Butterfly:* Orientalism, Gender, and a Critique of Essentialist Identity," *Cultural Critique* 16 (1990): 5–29; Gina Marchetti, *Romance and the "Yellow Peril": Race, Sex, and Discursive Strategies in Hollywood Fiction* (Berkeley: University of California Press, 1993); James S. Moy, "David Henry Hwang's *M. Butterfly* and Philip Kan Gotanda's *Yankee Dawg You Die:* Repositioning Chinese American Marginality on the American Stage," *Theater Journal* 42, no.1 (1990): 48–56; and Karen Shimakawa, "Who's to Say? Or, Making Space for Gender and Ethnicity in *M. Butterfly*," *Theatre Journal* 45, no. 3 (1993): 349–62.

5. At the time I created the performance version of "The Amazing Chinese American Acrobat," I was codirecting the Rad Asian Sisters with Los Angeles–based performance artist Denise Uyehara. Uyehara founded the group in 1997 as an ongoing performance and writing workshop for Asian and Asian American women; it has since become a co-gendered organization. An ongoing dilemma was how to direct work and give feedback to artists who joined the group because it was identified as a space for Asian American women, without essentializing the subject position of Asian American women.

6. See Lisa Lowe for a discussion of the aesthetics of resistance, as an example of how Asian American literary scholars write against canonical understandings of what constitutes great literature: *Immigrant Acts: On Asian American Cultural Politics* (Durham, N.C.: Duke University Press, 1996).

7. Dorinne Kondo and Karen Shimakawa recuperate Hwang from Moy's criticism by focusing primarily on the possibilities offered by the narrative content.

8. *Wu shu* is a choreographed Chinese martial art. Much of what is performed in contemporary martial arts films (e.g., Ang Lee's *Crouching Tiger, Hidden Dragon* [2000]) is *wu shu*. *Wu shu* competitions emphasize the performed aesthetics of choreographed forms, rather than self-defense.

9. "Performing Cultural Interventions: Community and Asian American Theater," conference panel at the 2001 Asian American Studies Conference, Toronto.

10. The publication of Esther Kim Lee's *A History of Asian American Theatre* (Cambridge: Cambridge University Press, 2006) gives shape to a canon for Asian American theater.

11. Dan Bacalzo, "Collective Autobiographies: The Process of Peeling," paper presented at the Association for Asian American Studies Conference, 31 March 2001, Toronto, Ontario; Priya Srinivasan, "South Asian Cultural Performances: Inscribing Identities on the Diasporic Bodies," paper presented at the Congress on Research and Dance, 4 December 1999, Pomona, California.

4. Mapping Membership: Class, Ethnicity, and the Making of *Stories from a Nail Salon*

1. Sukanya Rahman, *Dancing in the Family* (Delhi, India: Harper Collins, 2001).

2. Marta Savigliano, *Angora Matta: Fatal Acts of North-South Translation* (Middletown, Conn.: Wesleyan University Press, 2003).

3. Esther Kim Lee, *A History of Asian American Theatre* (Cambridge: Cambridge University Press, 2006).

4. The set of *Laughter from the Children of War* was made out of newspaper. If no one remembered to bring large amounts of newspaper to a performance, someone would be sent out to find it.

5. José Eduardo Limón, *Dancing with the Devil: Society and Cultural Poetics in Mexican American South Texas* (Madison: University of Wisconsin Press, 1994), 141; Yvonne Daniel, *Rumba: Dance and Social Change in Contemporary Cuba* (Bloomington: Indiana University Press, 1995), 21.

6. The term "refugee" is not only applied to Vietnamese Americans, but to Laotian and Cambodian Americans as well.

7. Considered one of the pioneers in Asian American performance, Nobuko Miyamoto was trained as a singer and dancer. She began her performing career in the 1950s, dancing in such Broadway productions as *Flower Drum Song, The King and I*, and *West Side Story*. After working on a docudrama about the Black Panther Party, Miyamoto was introduced to the Asian American movement and became interested in the intersection between art and politics. In 1978, Miyamoto founded Great Leap, one of the first Asian American performance art organizations established in the United States.

8. Jude Narita, *Walk the Mountain*, performance, Highways Performance Space, Santa Monica, California, 2002.

9. As quoted by Michelle Woo in "What's It Like to Work with Fingers and Toes?" Nguoi Viet 2 Online, 12 February 2004; http://nguoi-viet.com/absolutenm/anmviewer.asp?a=705&z=43. Accessed 15 December 2007.

10. Tara Bui, "Inside the Vietnamese Nail Salon," Nguoi Viet 2 Online, 5 April 2007; http://www.nguoi-viet.com/absolutenm/anmviewer.asp?a=57995&z=43. Accessed 15 December 2007.

5. Writing *Nail Salon*

1. Athough I consider the entire work choreographed—in the sense that all sections of the piece use movement—some of the scenes feature choreographed movement as their central mode of performance.

2. See chapter 6 for an in-depth discussion of The Engineer's American Dream and of Miss Chinatown.

3. These observations are based on conversations with Club O' Noodles members who interviewed people working in nail salons with predominantly African American clientele. One of the reasons the company undertook the project had to do with the extent to which the racial attitudes of Asian immigrants toward African Americans continues to mirror the dominant discourse of White racism.

4. After the Vietnam War, the government passed legislation to aid in the reunification of orphaned Amerasian children with their American fathers. Since mixed-race children, particularly those fathered by African American soldiers, were abandoned by Vietnamese mothers, U.S. officials often determined a child's eligibility for U.S. citizenship based on skin color, hair color, nose shape, and other visual differences among categories of "Whiteness," "Blackness," and "Asian-ness." The assumption that one can determine nationality based on visible racial difference assumes that the body of a mixed-raced subject can be dissected into individually discernible racial attributes.

5. I address this in more depth in chapter 6.

6. Pedagogy of the Scantily Clad:
Studying Miss Saigon in the Twenty-first Century

1. The *Miss Saigon* performed in 1999 at Theatre Royal Drury Lane in London had a flyer advertisement titled "You'll Miss Saigon" that included these quotes: "A piece of total theatre" (*Evening Standard*); "This tremendous musical set in Vietnam. It even has a helicopter landing on stage, but also a biting political message. Seriously exciting" (*Sunday Times,* 4 July 1999); and "A triumph and shattering experience . . . moves one to tears and also fills the heart to burst" (*Daily Mail*).

2. This is a reminder that the Asian American community is not just ethnically diverse, but politically diverse as well. Not all Asian Americans view stereotypes and social inequality with the same lens. While racist representations of Asian men may be objectionable to this man, seeing Asian women dancing in bikinis may not be objectionable to him. Rather than reading the performance as an atrocious representation of Asian women, he enjoyed the opportunity to visually consume the women's bodies from the point of view of a heterosexual male.

3. For a more recent contribution to the body of critical literature on *Miss Saigon* see Celine Parreñas Shimizu, "The Bind of Representation: Performing and Consuming Hypersexuality in *Miss Saigon,*" *Theatre Journal* 57, no. 2 (May 2005): 247–65. In *A History of Asian American Theatre* (Cambridge: Cambridge University Press, 2006) Esther Kim Lee provides a historical chronology of events leading up to the protest by Asian American members of Actor's Equity over the casting of a White actor, Jona-

than Pryce, in the lead role of The Engineer, which was written as an Eurasian character.

4. "Miss Saigon Soon in RP," *Manila Mail Bayanihan*, December 2000: B5.

5. Vernon Loeb, "U.S. Accused of Using Race to Target China Spy Suspect," *Los Angeles Times,* 17 August 1999: A17.

6. *A. Magazine* (June/July 2001): 14.

7. Kathy Walter, "Spotlight Students Become Pioneers in Musical Theater," *Your North Hills*, 18 April 2007, www.yournorthhills.com/node/1745; accessed April 18, 2007. Walter credits St. Joseph Regional High School's world high school premiere for bringing *Miss Saigon* into the repertory of high school theater programs. The list of schools following in the footsteps of St. Joseph includes Spotlight Performance Arts Academy in Pittsburgh, Pennsylvania; Huntington Beach Performing Arts Academy in Huntington Beach, California (2007), and West Aurora High School in Chicago, Illinois (2007). Linda Giardi, "West High's 'Miss Saigon' Named a Showstopper in USA Weekend Contest," *Beacon News*, 10 August 2007, http://www.suburbanchicago news.com/beaconnews/news/504943,2_1_AU10_WESTPLAY_S1.article; accessed August 10, 2007; Callie Prendiville, "Miss Saigon," *Orange County Register,* 27 March 2007, http://www.ocregister.com/ocregister/life/education/cappies/article_1632646 .php; accessed March 28, 2007.

8. Dorinne Kondo, "Art, Activism, Asia, Asian Americans," in *About Face: Performing Race in Fashion and Theater* (New York: Routledge, 1997), 227–57; Josephine Lee, "The Seduction of the Stereotype," in *Performing Asian America: Race and Ethnicity on the Contemporary Stage* (Philadelphia: Temple University Press, 1997), 91; Angela Pao, "The Eyes of the Storm: Gender, Genre and Cross-Casting in *Miss Saigon*," *Text and Performance Quarterly* 12 (January 1992): 21–39; Karen Shimakawa, " 'I'll be here . . . right where you left me': Mimetic Abjection/Mimetic Mimicry," in *National Abjection: The Asian American Body Onstage* (Durham, N.C.: Duke University Press, 2002), 99–128; Esther Kim Lee, "The *Miss Saigon* Controversy," in *A History of Asian American Theatre* (Cambridge: Cambridge University Press, 2006), 177–99.

9. Kondo "Art, Activism." Kondo chronicles the efforts which Asian American activists made to protest the Los Angeles opening of *Miss Saigon* and includes the unedited text of an editorial written for the *Los Angeles Times*. See also Yoko Yoshikawa, "The Heat is on *Miss Saigon* Coalition: Organizing across Race and Sexuality," in *The State of Asian America: Activism and Resistance in the 1990s*, ed. Karin Aguilar-San Juan (Boston: South End Press, 1994), 275–94.

10. Marina Heung, "The Family Romance of Orientalism: From *Madame Butterfly* to *Indochine*," in *Visions of the East: Orientalism in Film,* ed. Matthew Bernstein and Gaylyn Studlar (New Brunswick, N.J.: Rutgers University Press, 1997), 158–83.

11. I am using the term "White liberalism" to describe a notion of social safety, in

which White society or a portion of White society believes itself to be invested in undoing racism for the good of all people. Moving White liberalism from the margins to the center is not necessarily a shift in ideology, since Whiteness still maintains the center. Rather than overtly pushing away the margins, White liberalism expands to subsume fellow dissenters (especially people of color) and represent the most universally rational and applicable viewpoints. Thus, Whiteness can maintain its center while maintaining a hold on progressive politics. Since it is "progressive," it therefore cannot be discriminatory, and, thus, those that claim White liberalism is not enough are overly sensitive, have no sense of humor, and need to get over their victim mentality. White liberalism is not specific to White people, but describes a feeling of complacency and relative safety regardless of one's gender, race, sexuality, and religious and/or political affiliation. The term "equal opportunity employer" can be viewed as a weapon for White liberalism to defend itself against charges of discrimination. Because antidiscriminatory policies are articulated in great detail and are something rational people do not argue against, White liberalism operates as a political median for people to use as a measure for tolerance. Antidiscriminatory and antipreferential policies are promises made for a neutral present and future that will not be linked to sociopolitical or socioeconomic contexts.

12. David Henry Hwang's revival of *Flower Drum Song* opened in 2001 to sold-out audiences at the Ahmanson Theatre in Los Angeles, before opening on Broadway at the Virginia Theatre on October 17, 2002. The musical closed after 169 performances. *Flower Drum Song* was a revival of Rodgers and Hammerstein's adaptation of C. Y. Lee's book of the same name. Some audiences might have been familiar with the film version produced in 1961, which, like the original stage version, featured an all–Asian American cast. It is interesting to note that a large percentage of the 2001 cast of *Flower Drum Song* were veterans of *Miss Saigon* productions.

13. Fei-lan Pai's "Singing across the Pacific" examines the marketing of *Miss Saigon* to Asian audiences, in which the Asian press downplayed the musical's relationship to both *Madama Butterfly* and Vietnam. Pai argues that the musical's success is couched in an emphasis on fiction. "Singing across the Pacific: *Miss Saigon* and *Making Tracks*," master's thesis, University of Illinois–Urbana-Champaign, 2007.

14. Peter Royston and Sarah Schlesinger, *"Miss Saigon" Study Guide*, ed. Helen Sneed. (New York: Music Theatre International, 2000).

Big League Productions has taken down the official Web site for the 2002–2005 North American tour of *Miss Saigon*. In its place is a page that lists over forty quotes describing how the touring version is even better than the original (http://www.bigleague .org/high_saigon.htm; accessed April 5, 2009). A parent of an actor named Maddie, cast in the role of Tam for the 2000 spring/summer national tour, created a Web site which included a downloadable copy of the study guide (http://www.maddiesadventure .com/index.htm; accessed April 5, 2009). The official Web site of the U.K. national tour includes a section on educational resources with a different set of study guides asking similar questions (http://www.miss-saigon.com/educa tional/index.htm; accessed April 5, 2009).

15. Walter, "Spotlight Students Become Pioneers in Musical Theater," 18 April 2007, www.yournorthhills.com/node/1745.

16. Royston and Schlesinger, *"Miss Saigon" Study Guide*, 8.

17. Kondo, "Art, Activism."

18. Jonathan Burton, "New York Thirsty for Broadway Success," *Christian Science Monitor*, 22 August 1990: 9.

19. Joe Piedrafite, "The Last Night of the World: *Miss Saigon* Lands in Amherst," *Daily Collegian*, 13 October 2005, http://www.dailycollegian.com/vnews/display.v?Target; Tanya Manus, "Review: *Miss Saigon* Ends with a Bold Finish," *Rapid City Journal*, 15 October 2005, http://www.rapidcityjournal.com/articles/2005/10/15/entertainment; and Sarah D'Esti Miller, "*Miss Saigon* Star Savors the Honesty of Live Theater," *Press and Sun-Bulletin*, 13 October 2005, http://www.pressconnects.com/entertainment/stories; all accessed October 15, 2007.

20. William A. Henry, "Memories of a World on Fire," *Time*, 22 April 1991: 91.

21. In Edward Behr and Mark Steyn, *The Story of "Miss Saigon"* (New York: Arcade, 1991), 18.

22. Ibid.

23. Behr and Steyn, *The Story of "Miss Saigon,"* 22.

24. Ibid.

25. Behr and Steyn, *The Story of "Miss Saigon,"* 23.

26. Ibid.

27. Behr and Steyn, *The Story of "Miss Saigon,"* 26.

28. For another reading of the photograph, see Heung, "The Family Romance of Orientalism." Heung discusses in detail the significance of the photograph as a proscription for foregrounding Asian maternal sacrifice and as a way of recuperating the ambiguities of masculinity and paternity in the post–Vietnam War United States.

29. Behr and Steyn, *The Story of "Miss Saigon,"* 26.

30. Ibid., 30.

31. Ibid.

32. Behr and Steyn, *The Story of "Miss Saigon,"* 188.

33. The Engineer is written as an "Eurasian" character, but for all purposes in the musical he is portrayed as a Vietnamese man who happens to have a French father (whom he has never met). The writers and producer considered The Engineer the "perfect" role to cast, since either a Caucasian or an Asian could play him, until the controversy in the United States threatened to cancel the show on Broadway.

34. Behr and Steyn, *The Story of "Miss Saigon,"* 15.

35. Ibid.

36. Ibid.

37. Ibid., 16.

38. Renny Christopher, *The Viet Nam War / The American War: Images and Representations in Euro-American and Vietnamese American Exile Narratives* (Amherst: University of Massachusetts Press, 1995).

39. " 'The Engineer,' Schönberg said, 'must be like a sneaky little Oriental mouse at this point.' " Behr and Steyn, *The Story of "Miss Saigon,"* 166.

40. Royston and Schlesinger, *"Miss Saigon" Study Guide*, 18.

41. Behr and Steyn, *The Story of "Miss Saigon,"* 11–12.

42. Gayatri Spivak as cited in Traise Yamamoto, *Masking Selves, Making Subjects: Japanese American Women, Identity, and the Body* (Berkeley: University of California Press, 1999), 25.

43. Behr and Steyn, *The Story of "Miss Saigon,"* 13–14.

44. Katherine H. S. Moon, *Sex Among Allies: Military Prostitution in U.S.-Korea Relations* (New York: Columbia University Press, 1997).

45. Behr and Steyn, *The Story of "Miss Saigon,"* 14.

46. Yamamoto, *Masking Selves*, 25.

47. Royston and Schlesinger, *"Miss Saigon" Study Guide*, 18.

48. Yamamoto, *Masking Selves*, 96.

49. Eugenia Kaw, "Medicalization of Racial Features: Asian American Women and Cosmetic Surgery," *Medical Anthropology Quarterly* 7, no. 1 (1993): 74–89; quoted in Yamamoto.

50. "Senators' Memories," *NewsHour with Jim Lehrer*, PBS, 2 May 2000.

51. Ibid.

52. Behr and Steyn, *The Story of "Miss Saigon,"* 156–57.

53. Jonathan Van Meter, "Broadway Baby," *Vogue* (June 1991): 178.

54. Ibid., 182.

55. Behr and Steyn, *The Story of "Miss Saigon,"* 127.

56. Van Meter, "Broadway Baby," 220.

57. Behr and Steyn, *The Story of "Miss Saigon,"* 14.

BIBLIOGRAPHY

Agamben, Giorgio. *The Coming Community*. Translated by Michael Hardt. Minneapolis: University of Minnesota Press, 1993.

Aguilar-San Juan, Karin, ed. *The State of Asian America: Activism and Resistance in the 1990s*. Boston: South End Press, 1994.

Albright, Ann Cooper. *Choreographing Difference: The Body and Identity in Contemporary Dance*. Hanover, N.H.: University Press of New England, 1997.

Alexander, Garth. "Japanese Take *Saigon* to Heart." *Variety,* 18 May 1992: 65.

Allen, Virginia M. *The Femme Fatale: Erotic Icon*. New York: Whitson, 1983.

Althusser, Louis. *Lenin and Philosophy and Other Essays*. Translated by Ben Brewster. New York: Monthly Review Press, 1971.

Anderegg, Michael, ed. *Inventing Vietnam: The War in Film and Television*. Philadelphia: Temple University Press, 1991.

Anderson, Benedict. *Imagined Communities*. London: Verso, 1983.

"Announcement on *Miss Saigon* Expected Today." *New York Times,* 21 August 1990: C14.

Anzaldúa, Gloria. *Borderlands: La Frontera a New Mestiza*. San Francisco: Aunt Lute Foundation Books, 1987.

Asian Women United of California, eds. *Making Waves: An Anthology of Writings by and about Asian American Women*. Boston: Beacon Press, 1989.

Au, Susan. *Ballet and Modern Dance*. London: Thames and Hudson, 1988.

Bacalzo, Dan. "Collective Autobiographies: The Process of Peeling." Conference paper. Association for Asian American Studies Conference. Toronto, Ontario, 31 March 2001.

Backscheider, Paula R. *Spectacular Politics: Theatrical Power and Mass Culture in Early Modern England*. Baltimore, Md.: Johns Hopkins University Press, 1993.

"Bad Show from Actors' Equity." Editorial. *Los Angeles Times,* 10 August 1990: B6.

Banes, Sally. *Dancing Women: Female Bodies on Stage*. New York: Routledge, 1998.

——. *Democracy's Body: Judson Dance Theater, 1962–1964*. Durham, N.C.: Duke University Press, 1993.

——. *Terpsichore in Sneakers: Post-Modern Dance*. 2nd ed. Middletown, Conn.: Wesleyan University Press, 1987.

——. *Writing Dancing: In the Age of Postmodernism*. Hanover, N.H.: University Press of New England, 1994.

Barkan, Elazar, and Marie-Denise Shelton, eds. *Borders, Exiles, Diasporas*. Stanford, Calif.: Stanford University Press, 1998.

Barmé, Geremie R. *In the Red: On Contemporary Chinese Culture*. New York: Columbia University Press, 1999.

Barthes, Roland. *Empire of Signs*. 1970. Translated by Richard Howard. New York: Hill and Wang, 1982.

———. *Mythologies*. 1957. Translated by Annette Lavers. York, England: The Noonday Press, 1972.

Baudrillard, Jean. *America*. 1986. Translated by Chris Turner. London: Verso, 1988.

———. *For a Critique of the Political Economy of the Sign*. Translated by Charles Levin. New York: Telos Press, 1981.

Beaufort, John. "*Miss Saigon* a True Stage Spectacle." Review of *Miss Saigon*, music by Claude-Michel Schönberg, book by Alain Boublil and Claude-Michel Schönberg, lyrics by Alain Boublil and Richard Maltby Jr. Broadway Theatre, New York. *Christian Science Monitor,* 22 April 1991: 11.

Becker, Carol, ed. *The Subversive Imagination: Artists, Society, and Social Responsibility*. New York: Routledge, 1994.

Behr, Edward, and Mark Steyn. *The Story of Miss Saigon*. New York: Arcade, 1991.

Belmar, Sima. "Boxed In: The Nature of Nature Is Trapped in Stereotypes." *San Francisco Bay Guardian,* 21–27 March 2001: 49.

Berlant, Lauren. "National Brands/National Body: Imitation of Life." In *Comparative American Identities: Race, Sex, and Nationality in the Modern Text,* edited by Hortense J. Spillers, 110–40. New York: Routledge, 1991.

———. *The Queen of America Goes to Washington City: Essays on Sex and Citizenship*. Durham, N.C.: Duke University Press, 1997.

Bernstein, Matthew, and Gaylyn Studlar, eds. *Visions of the East: Orientalism in Film*. New Brunswick, N.J.: Rutgers University Press, 1997.

Bernstein, Richard. "The Arts Catch Up with a Society in Disarray." *New York Times,* 2 September 1990, sec. 2, p. 1+.

Berson, Misha. *Between Worlds: Contemporary Asian-American Plays*. New York: Theatre Communications Group, 1990.

"Best of 1991 Theater." *Time,* 6 January 1992: 78.

Bhabha, Homi K. "The Other Question: Difference, Discrimination and the Discourse of Colonialism." 1986. In *Out There: Marginalization and Contemporary Cultures,* edited by Russell Ferguson, Martha Gever, Trinh T. Minh-ha, and Cornel West, 71–87. Cambridge, Mass.: MIT Press, 1990.

"Biz Slips: *Cyrano* $116g." *Variety,* 7 March 1994: 66.

Boal, Augusto. *Theatre of the Oppressed*. 1974. Translated by Charles A. and Maria-Odilia Leal McBride. New York: Theatre Communications Group, 1985.

Boyarin, Jonathan, ed. *Remapping Memory: The Politics of TimeSpace*. Minneapolis: University of Minnesota Press, 1994.

Brossard, Nicole. *Picture Theory*. New York: Roof Books, 1990.

Brustein, Robert. "Lighten Up, America." *New Republic* (10–17 September 1991): 35+.

———. "The Use and Abuse of Multiculturalism." *New Republic* (16–23 September 1991): 31–34.

Bui, Tara. "Inside the Vietnamese Nail Salon." Nguoi Viet 2 Online (5 April 2007), http://nguoi-viet.com/absolutenm/anmviewer.asp?a=57995.

Burgoyne, Robert. "National Identity, Gender Identity, and the 'Rescue Fantasy' in *Born on the Fourth of July*." *Screen* 35, no. 3 (1994): 211–43.

Burt, Ramsay. *Alien Bodies: Representations of Modernity, Race and Nation in Early Modern Dance*. New York: Routledge, 1998.

———. "Dance Theory, Sociology, and Aesthetics." *Dance Research Journal* 32, no. 1 (2000): 125–30.

———. *The Male Dancer: Bodies, Spectacle, Sexualities*. New York: Routledge, 1995.

Burton, Jonathan. "New York Thirsty for Broadway Success." *Christian Science Monitor,* 22 August 1990: 8.

Butler, Judith. *Bodies that Matter: On the Discursive Limits of "Sex."* New York: Routledge, 1993.

———. *Gender Trouble: Feminism and the Subversion of Identity*. New York: Routledge, 1990.

Caldwell, Helen. *The Dancer and the Dances*. Berkeley: University of California Press, 1977.

Carrier, James G., ed. *Occidentalism: Images of the West*. Oxford: Clarendon Press, 1995.

Carter, Alexandra, ed. *The Routledge Dance Studies Reader*. New York: Routledge, 1998.

Case, Sue-Ellen. *The Domain-Matrix: Performing Lesbian at the End of Print Culture*. Bloomington: Indiana University Press, 1996.

Case, Sue-Ellen, Philip Brett, and Susan Leigh Foster, eds. *Cruising the Performative: Interventions into the Representation of Ethnicity, Nationality, and Sexuality*. Bloomington: Indiana University Press, 1995.

Case, Sue-Ellen, and Janelle Reinelt, eds. *The Performance of Power: Theatrical Discourse and Politics*. Iowa City: University of Iowa Press, 1991.

Chang, Tisa, and Dominick Balletta. Letter. "Actors' Equity Had to Fight Over *Miss Saigon*." *New York Times,* 10 August 1990: A24.

Chatterjea, Ananya. *Butting Out: Reading the Resistive Choreographies Through Works by Jawole Willa Jo Zollar and Chandralekha*. Middletown, Conn.: Wesleyan University Press, 2004.

Cherniavsky, Felix. *The Salome Dancer: The Life and Times of Maud Allan*. Toronto: McClelland and Stewart, 1991.

Chong, Ping, and Muna Tseng. "Slut For Art." In *Tokens? The NYC Asian American*

Experience on Stage, edited by Alvin Eng, 378–405. New York: Asian American Writers Workshop, 1999.

Chow, Rey. *Ethics After Idealism: Theory, Culture, Ethnicity, Reading*. Bloomington: Indiana University Press, 1998.

———. *Woman and Chinese Modernity: The Politics of Reading Between West and East*. Minneapolis: University of Minnesota Press, 1991.

———. *Writing Diaspora: Tactics of Intervention in Contemporary Cultural Studies*. Bloomington: Indiana University Press, 1993.

Christopher, Renny. *The Viet Nam War / The American War: Images and Representations in Euro-American and Vietnamese Exile Narratives*. Amherst: University of Massachusetts Press, 1995.

Chun, Allen. "Fuck Chineseness: On the Ambiguities of Ethnicity as Culture as Identity." *Boundary* 23, no. 2 (1996): 111–38.

Cixous, Hélène. *Three Steps on the Ladder of Writing*. Translated by Sarah Cornell and Susan Sellers. New York: Columbia University Press, 1993.

Clément, Catherine. *Opera: Or the Undoing of Women*. 1979. Translated by Betsy Wing. Minneapolis: University of Minnesota Press, 1988.

Clifford, James. "On Ethnographic Authority." In *Predicament of Culture: Twentieth-Century Ethnography, Literature, and Art*, 21–54. Cambridge, Mass.: Harvard University Press, 1988.

———. *Routes: Travel and Translation in the Late Twentieth Century*. Cambridge, Mass.: Harvard University Press, 1997.

Corliss, Richard. "Will Broadway *Miss Saigon?*" *Time*, 20 August 1990: 75.

Cowan, Jane. *Dance and the Body Politic in Northern Greece*. Princeton, N.J.: Princeton University Press, 1990.

Crary, Jonathan, and Sanford Kwinter, eds. *Zone: Incorporations*. New York: Zone, 1992.

Crenshaw, Kimberlé, Neil Gotanda, Gary Peller, and Kendall Thomas, eds. *Critical Race Theory: The Key Writings that Formed the Movement*. Foreword by Cornel West. New York: New York Press, 1995.

Daly, Ann. "The Balanchine Woman: Of Hummingbirds and Channel Swimmers." *Drama Review* 31, no. 1 (1987): 8–21.

———. *Done into Dance: Isadora Duncan in America*. Bloomington: Indiana University Press, 1995.

Dalva, Nancy. "DanceTheater: Broadway Winners." Review of *Miss Saigon*, music by Claude-Michel Schönberg, book by Alain Boublil and Claude-Michel Schönberg, lyrics by Alain Boublil and Richard Maltby Jr. Broadway Theatre, New York. *Dance Magazine* (August 1991): 53.

Daniel, Yvonne. *Rumba: Dance and Social Change in Contemporary Cuba*. Bloomington: Indiana University Press, 1995.

de Certeau, Michel. *The Practice of Everyday Life*. Translated by Steven Randall. Berkeley: University of California Press, 1984.

——. *The Writing of History*. 1975. Translated by Tom Conley. New York: Columbia University Press, 1988.

DeConde, Alexander. *Ethnicity, Race, and American Foreign Policy: A History*. Boston: Northeastern University Press, 1992.

Debord, Guy. *The Society of the Spectacle*. Translated by Donald Nicholson-Smith. New York: Zone Books, 1995.

De Frantz, Thomas. *Dancing Revelations: Alvin Ailey's Embodiment of African American Culture*. New York: Oxford University Press, 2004.

De Lauretis, Teresa. *Alice Doesn't: Feminism, Semiotics, Cinema*. Bloomington: Indiana University Press, 1984.

Deleuze, Giles, and Felix Guattari. "Introduction: Rhizome." In *A Thousand Plateaus: Capitalism and Schizophrenia*. 1980. Translated by Brian Massumi. Minneapolis: University of Minnesota Press, 1987.

Delgado, Celeste Fraser, and José Esteban Muñoz, eds. *Every-Night Life: Culture and Dance in Latin/o America*. Durham, N.C.: Duke University Press, 1997.

Derrida, Jacques. *Limited Inc*. 1977. Evanston, Ill.: Northwestern University Press, 1988.

Desmond, Jane. "Dancing Out the Difference: Cultural Imperialism and Ruth St. Denis' 'Radha' of 1906." *Signs* 17, no. 1 (1991): 28–49.

——, ed. *Meaning in Motion: New Cultural Studies of Dance*. Durham, N.C.: Duke University Press, 1997.

De Vries, Hillary. "From the Paris Sewers to Vietnam's Streets." *New York Times,* 17 September 1989, sec. 2, p. 5+.

Diamond, Elin, ed. *Performance and Cultural Politics*. New York: Routledge, 1996.

Disch, Thomas M. Review of *Miss Saigon*, music by Claude-Michel Schönberg, book by Alain Boublil and Claude-Michel Schönberg, lyrics by Alain Boublil and Richard Maltby, Jr. Broadway Theatre, New York. *Nation* (13 May 1991): 642–44.

Donohue, Maura, "From 'When You're Old Enough.'" In *Watermark: Vietnamese American Poetry and Prose*, edited by Barbara Tran, Monique T. D. Truong, and Luu Truong Khoi, 105–10. New York: Asian American Writers Workshop, 1998.

Dunning, Jennifer. "Miss Saigon Proposal Is Being Negotiated." *New York Times,* 13 December 1990: C18.

Dyer, Richard. *The Matter of Images: Essays on Representations*. London: Routledge, 1993.

——. *White*. London: Routledge, 1997.

Eng, Alvin, ed. *Tokens? The NYC Asian American Experience on Stage*. New York: Asian American Writers Workshop, 1999.

Eng, David L. "In the Shadows of the Diva: Committing Homosexuality in David Henry Hwang's *M. Butterfly*." *Amerasia Journal* 20, no. 1 (1994): 93–116.

Erlmann, Veit. *Nightsong: Performance, Power, and Practice in South Africa*. Chicago: University of Chicago Press, 1996.

Espiritu, Yen Le. *Asian American Women and Men: Labor, Laws, and Love*. Thousand Oaks, Calif.: Sage, 1997.

Evans, Greg. "Winter Chills: Empty Seats at Empty Fables." *Variety*, 7 March 1992: 65+.

Fabian, Johannes. *Power and Performance: Ethnographic Explorations through Proverbial Wisdom and Theater in Shaba, Zaïre*. Madison: University of Wisconsin Press, 1990.

——. "Presence and Representation (1990)." In *Time and the Work of Anthropology: Critical Essays 1971–1991*, 207–24. Chur, Switzerland: Harwood Academic Publishers, 1991.

——. *Time and the Other: How Anthropology Makes Its Object*. New York: Columbia University Press, 1983.

Fanon, Frantz. *Black Skin, White Masks*. New York: Grove Press, 1967.

Fine, Michelle, Lois Weis, Linda C. Powell, and L. Mun Wong, eds. *Off White: Readings on Race, Power, and Society*. New York: Routledge, 1997.

Fisher, Jennifer. *Nutcracker Nation: How an Old World Ballet Became a Christmas Tradition in the New World*. New Haven, Conn.: Yale University Press, 2004.

Foster, Susan L, ed. *Choreographing History*. Bloomington: Indiana University Press, 1995.

——, ed. *Corporealities: Dancing Knowledge, Culture and Power*. New York: Routledge, 1996.

——. "Dancing Bodies." In *Zone: Incorporations,* edited by Jonathan Crary and Sanford Kwinter, 480–96. New York: Zone, 1992.

——. *Reading Dancing*. Berkeley: University of California Press, 1986.

Foucault, Michel. *The Archaeology of Knowledge and the Discourse on Language*. 1969. Translated by A. M. Sheridan Smith. New York: Pantheon Books, 1972.

——. *Discipline and Punish: The Birth of the Prison*. 1975. Translated by Alan Sheridan. New York: Vintage Books, 1979.

——. *The Order of Things: An Archaeology of the Human Sciences*. 1966. New York: Vintage Books, 1994.

Foulkes, Julia. *Modern Bodies*. Chapel Hill: University of North Carolina Press, 2002.

Franko, Mark. *Dancing Modernism/Performing Politics*. Bloomington: Indiana University Press, 1995.

Full Metal Jacket. Directed by Stanly Kubrick. Warner Brothers, 1987.

Fung, Richard. "Call in the Tropes!: *Miss Saigon* Undergoes Analysis." *Fuse* (Winter 1993–94): 7+.

Furman, Frida Kerner. *Facing the Mirror: Older Women and Beauty Shop Culture*. New York: Routledge, 1997.

Fusco, Coco. *English is Broken Here: Notes on Cultural Fusion in the Americas*. New York: New York Press, 1995.

Gates Jr., Henry Louis, ed. *"Race," Writing, and Difference*. Chicago: University of Chicago Press, 1985.

Geertz, Clifford. "Thick Description: Toward an Interpretive Theory of Culture." In *The Interpretation of Cultures: Selected Essays*, 3–30. New York: Basic Books, 1973.

Gest, T., and D. L. Boroughs. "Caste in Casting on Broadway." *U.S. News & World Report*, 20 August 1990: 13.

Giardi, Linda. "West High's 'Miss Saigon' Named a Showstopper in USA Weekend Contest," *Beacon News*, 10 August 2007, http://www.suburbanchicagonews.com/ beaconnews/ news/504943,2_1_AU10_WESTPLAY_S1.article.

Goellner, Ellen W., and Jacqueline Shea Murphy, eds. *Bodies of the Text: Dance as Theory, Literature as Dance*. New Brunswick, N.J.: Rutgers University Press, 1994.

Goldberg, David Theo, ed. *Anatomy of Racism*. Minneapolis: University of Minnesota Press, 1990.

Gooding-Williams, Robert. *Reading Rodney King: Reading Urban Uprising*. New York: Routledge, 1993.

Gottschild, Brenda Dixon. *Digging the Africanist Presence in African American Performance: Dance and Other Contexts*. Westport, Conn.: Greenwood Press, 1996.

——. "Some Thoughts on Choreographing History." In *Meaning in Motion: New Cultural Studies of Dance*, edited by Jane C. Desmond, 167–77. Durham, N.C.: Duke University Press, 1997.

Goux, Jean-Joseph. *Symbolic Economies: After Marx and Freud*. 1973. Translated by Jennifer Curtiss Gage. Ithaca, N.Y.: Cornell University Press, 1990.

Graff, Ellen. *Stepping Left: Dance and Politics in New York City, 1928–1942*. Durham, N.C.: Duke University Press, 1997.

Graham, Lawrence Otis. *Our Kind of People: Inside America's Black Upper Class*. New York: Harper, 1999.

Granville, Kari, and Don Shirley. "Actors' Equity Says White Can Portray Eurasian." *Los Angeles Times*, 17 August 1990: A4.

Green, Richard C. "(Up)Staging the Primitive: Pearl Primus and the 'Negro Problem' in American Dance." In *Dancing Many Drums: Excavations in African American Dance*, edited by Thomas F. DeFrantz, 105–42. Madison: University of Wisconsin Press, 2002.

Habermas, Jürgen. *The Structural Transformation of the Public Sphere: An Inquiry into a Category of Bourgeois Society*. 1962. Translated by Thomas Burger with the assistance of Frederick Lawrence. Cambridge, Mass.: MIT Press, 1991.

Hamamoto, Darrell Y. *Monitored Peril: Asian Americans and the Politics of TV Representation*. Minneapolis: University of Minnesota Press, 1994.

Hart, Lynda, and Peggy Phelan, eds. *Acting Out: Feminist Performances*. Ann Arbor: University of Michigan Press, 1993.

Henry, William A. "Does Color Blindness Count?" *Time* (27 August 1990): 67.

———. "Last Exit to the Land of Hope." *Time* (8 April 1991): 72–74.

———. "Memories of a World on Fire." *Time* (22 April 1991): 91.

Hering, Doris. Review of the Asian New Dance Coalition, Sun Ock Lee's Studio. *Dancemagazine* (July 1979): 106–8.

Hertzberg, Hendrik. "Washington Diarist: Actors' Inequity." *New Republic* (3 September 1990): 46.

Heung, Marina. "The Family Romance of Orientalism." In *Visions of the East: Orientalism in Film,* edited by Matthew Bernstein and Gaylyn Studlar, 158–83. New Brunswick, N.J.: Rutgers University Press, 1997.

Hing, Bill Ong. *Making and Remaking Asian America through Immigration Policy, 1850–1990*. Stanford, Calif.: Stanford University Press, 1993.

Hoare, Quintin, and Geoffrey Nowell Smith, eds. and trans. *Selections from the Prison Notebooks of Antonio Gramsci*. New York: International Publishers, 1971.

Houston, Velina Hasu. *The Politics of Life: Four Plays by Asian American Women*. Philadelphia: Temple University Press, 1993.

Hughes, Holly, and David Roman, eds. *O Solo Homo: The New Queer Performance*. New York: Grove Press, 1998.

Humphrey, Doris. *The Art of Making Dances*. New York: Grove Press, 1959.

Husman, J. K. *Against Nature*. 1884. Translated by Robert Baldick. London: Penguin Books, 1959.

"Inequity." *National Review* (3 September 1990): 15.

Innis, Robert E. *Semiotics: An Introductory Anthology*. Bloomington: Indiana University Press, 1985.

Iyer, Pico. "The Masks of Minority Terrorism." *Time* (3 September 1990): 86.

Jackson, Michael. *Paths Toward a Clearing: Radical Empiricism and Ethnographic Inquiry*. Bloomington: Indiana University Press, 1989.

Jameson, Fredric. *Postmodernism: Or the Cultural Logic of Late Capitalism*. Durham, N.C.: Duke University Press, 1991.

Joffee, Linda. "*Les Miz*' Team's New Musical Gets Warm Reception in London." *Christian Science Monitor,* 2 November 1989: 10.

———. "Next: *Miss Saigon*." *Christian Science Monitor,* 19 January 1989: 10.

———. "The Man behind Musical Hits." *Christian Science Monitor,* 22 April 1991: 10.

John, Nicholas, ed. *Madam Butterfly, Madama Butterfly Opera Guide 26*. London: John Calder Press, 1984.

Jones, Bill T. *Last Night on Earth*. With Peggy Gillespie. New York: Pantheon Books, 1995.

———. Introduction to *Continuous Replay: The Photographs of Arnie Zane*. Edited by Jonathan Green, 10–13. Cambridge, Mass.: MIT Press, 1999.

Kaw, Eugenia. "Medicalization of Racial Features: Asian American Women and Cosmetic Surgery." *Medical Anthropology Quarterly* 7, no. 1 (1993): 74–89.

Kealiinohomoku, Joann. "An Anthropologist Looks at Ballet as a Form of Ethnic Dance." In *Moving History/Dancing Cultures: A Dance Studies Reader*, edited by Ann Dils and Ann Cooper Albright, 33–43. Middletown, Conn.: Wesleyan University Press, 2001.

Kendall, Elizabeth. *Where She Danced*. New York: Alfred A. Knopf, 1979.

Kiernan, V. G. *Imperialism and Its Contradictions*. Edited and introduction by Harvey J. Kaye. New York: Routledge, 1995.

Kim, Kwang Chung. *Koreans in the Hood: Conflict with African Americans*. Baltimore, Md.: Johns Hopkins University Press, 1999.

King, Robert L. "Recent Drama." *Massachusetts Review* 32, no. 1 (1991): 150.

Kingston, Maxine Hong. *China Men*. New York: Vintage, 1977.

———. *Tripmaster Monkey: His Fake Book*. New York: Vintage, 1987.

———. *The Woman Warrior*. New York: Vintage, 1976.

Kirstein, Lincoln. *Dance: A Short History of Classic Theatrical Dancing*. New York: Greenwood Press, 1935.

Kondo, Dorinne K. *About Face: Performing Race in Fashion and Theater*. New York: Routledge, 1997.

———. *Crafting Selves: Power, Gender, and Discourses of Identity in a Japanese Workplace*. Chicago: University of Chicago Press, 1990.

———. "*M. Butterfly*: Orientalism, Gender, and a Critique of Essentialist Identity." *Cultural Critique* 16 (1990): 5–29.

Koritz, Amy. "Dancing the Orient for England: Maud Allan's 'The Vision of Salome.'" *Theatre Journal* 46, no. 1 (1994): 63–78.

Kreemer, Connie, ed. *Further Steps: Fifteen Choreographers on Modern Dance*. New York: Harper and Row, 1987.

Kurahashi, Yuko. *Asian American Culture on Stage: The History of the East West Players*. New York: Garland, 1999.

Lacan, Jacques. *Écrits: A Selection*. 1966. Translated by Alan Sheridan. New York: W. W. Norton, 1977.

Laclau, Ernesto, and Chantal Mouffe. *Hegemony and Socialist Strategy: Towards a Radical Democratic Politics*. London: Verso, 1985.

Lam, Andrew. "Love, Money, Prison, Sin, Revenge." *Los Angeles Times Magazine* (13 March 1994): 24–30, 56–58.

Lampert, Ellen. "*Miss Saigon*: A $10 Million Musical Import." *Theatre Crafts,* April 1991: 34+.

Larrain, Jorge. *Ideology and Cultural Identity: Modernity and the Third World Presence*. Cambridge: Polity Press, 1994.

Laughter from the Children of War. Directed by Hung Nguyen and Nobuko Miyamoto. University of California, Riverside. 16 May 1996.

Laughter from the Children of War. Directed by Hung Nguyen and Nobuko Miyamoto. Bowers Museum, Santa Ana, California. 26 January 1997.

Laughter from the Children of War. Directed by Hung Nguyen and Nobuko Miyamoto. Montgomery Theater, San Jose, California. 9 August 1997.

Lavie, Smadar, and Ted Swedenburg, eds. *Displacement, Diaspora, and Geographies of Identity*. Durham, N.C.: Duke University Press, 1996.

Lee, Esther Kim. *A History of Asian American Theatre*. Cambridge: Cambridge University Press, 2006.

Lee, Josephine. *Performing Asian America: Race and Ethnicity on the Contemporary Stage*. Philadelphia: Temple University Press, 1997.

Lee, Robert G. *Orientals: Asian Americans in Popular Culture*. Philadelphia: Temple University Press, 1999.

"Senators' Memories." *NewsHour with Jim Lehrer*. PBS, 2 May 2002.

Leong, Russell, ed. *Asian American Sexualities: Dimensions of the Gay and Lesbian Experience*. New York: Routledge, 1996.

——, ed. *Moving the Image: Independent Asian Pacific American Media Arts*. Los Angeles: UCLA Asian American Studies Center Press, 1991.

Lesschaeve, Jacqueline. *The Dancer and the Dance: Merce Cunningham in Conservation with Jacqueline Lesschaeve*. New York: Marion Boyars, 1985.

Levi-Strauss, Claude. *Tristes Tropiques*. 1955. Translated by John and Doreen Weightman. New York: Penguin Books, 1992.

Lewis, J. Lowell. *Ring of Liberation: Deceptive Discourse in Brazilian Capoeira*. Chicago: University of Chicago Press, 1992.

Lim-Hing, Sharon, ed. *The Very Inside: An Anthology of Writing by Asian And Pacific Islander Lesbian and Bisexual Women*. Toronto: Sister Vision Press, 1994.

Limón, José E. *Dancing With the Devil: Society and Cultural Poetics in Mexican-American South Texas*. Madison: University of Wisconsin Press, 1994.

Lippard, Lucy R., ed. *Mixed Blessings: New Art in a Multicultural America*. New York: Pantheon Books, 1990.

Loeb, Vernon. "U.S. Accused of Using Race to Target China Spy Suspect." *Los Angeles Times,* 17 August 1999: A17.

Lott, Eric. *Love and Theft: Blackface Minstrelsy and the American Working Class*. New York: Oxford University Press, 1993.

"Lost Courage, Lost Play." Editorial. *New York Times,* 9 August 1990: A22.

Lowe, Lisa. *Immigrant Acts*: *On Asian American Cultural Politics*. Durham, N.C.: Duke University Press, 1996.

Lum, Casey Man Kong. *In Search of a Voice: Karaoke and The Construction of Identity in Chinese America*. Mahwah, N.J.: Lawrence Erlbaum Associates, 1996.

Machida, Margo, ed. *Asia/America: Identities in Contemporary Asian American Art*. New York: Asia Society Galleries and The New Press, 1994.

MacLear, Kyo. "Sex, Lies and Stereotypes." *Art & Soul* (August 1993): 31+.

Maharidge, Dale. *The Coming White Minority: California, Multiculturalism, and America's Future*. New York: Vintage Books, 1996.

Maira, Sunaina. "Belly Dancing: Arab-Face, Orientalist Feminism and U.S. Empire." *American Quarterly* 60, no. 2 (June 2008): 317–45.

The Making of "Miss Saigon." A 54th Parallel Production for Thames Television. Prod. and dir. David Wright. VHS. New York: HBO Video, c. 1989.

Malone, Jacqui. *Stepping on the Blues: The Visible Rhythms of African American Dance*. Urbana: University of Illinois Press, 1996.

Manalansan IV, Martin F. "Cooking up the Senses: A Critical Embodied Approach to the Study of Food and Asian American Television Audience." In *Alien Encounters: Popular Culture in America*, edited by Mimi Thi Nguyen and Thuy Linh Nguyen Tu, 179–93. Durham, N.C.: Duke University Press, 2007.

——. "(Dis)Orienting the Body: Locating Symbolic Resistance among Filipino Gay Men." *Positions: East Asia Cultures Critique* 2 (Spring 1994): 73–90.

Manning, Susan. *Ecstasy and the Demon: Feminism and Nationalism in the Dances of Mary Wigman*. Berkeley: University of California Press, 1993.

——. *Modern Dance Negro Dance*. Minneapolis: University of Minnesota Press, 2004.

Manus, Tanya. "Review: *Miss Saigon* Ends with a Bold Finish." *Rapid City Journal,* 15 October 2005, http://www.rapidcityjournal.com/articles/2005/10/15/entertainment.

Marchetti, Gina. *Romance and the "Yellow Peril": Race, Sex, and Discursive Strategies in Hollywood Fiction*. Berkeley: University of California Press, 1993.

Marcus, George, ed. *Rereading Cultural Anthropology*. Durham, N.C.: Duke University Press, 1992.

Marks, Elaine, and Isabelle de Courtivron, eds. and intro. 1980. *New French Feminisms: An Anthology*. New York: Schocken Books, 1981.

Martin, Randy. "Agency and History: The Demands of Dance Ethnography." In *Choreographing History,* edited by Susan Leigh Foster, 105–15. Bloomington: Indiana University Press, 1995.

——. *Critical Moves: Dance Studies in Theory and Politics*. Durham, N.C.: Duke University Press, 1998.

——. *Performance as Political Act: The Embodied Self*. New York: Bergin and Garvey Publishers, 1990.

Mazumdar, Sucheta. "General Introduction: A Woman-Centered Perspective on Asian American History." In *Making Waves: An Anthology of Writings by and about Asian American Women*, edited by Asian Women United of California, 1–22. Boston: Beacon Press, 1989.

McLean, Adrienne L. "The Thousand Ways There Are to Move." In *Visions of the East: Orientalism in Film,* edited by Matthew Bernstein and Gaylyn Studlar, 130–57. New Brunswick, N.J.: Rutgers University Press, 1997.

Meltzer, Françoise. *Salome and the Dance of Writing: Portraits of Mimesis in Literature*. Chicago: University of Chicago Press, 1987.

Mercer, Kobena. "Black Hair/Style Politics." In *Out There: Marginalization and Contemporary Cultures,* edited by Russell Ferguson, Martha Gever, Trinh T. Minh-ha, and Cornel West, 247–64. Cambridge, Mass.: The MIT Press, 1990.

Michaelsen, Scott. *The Limits of Multiculturalism: Interrogating the Origins of American Anthropology*. Minneapolis: University of Minnesota Press, 1999.

Miller, D. A. *Bringing Out Barthes*. Berkeley: University of California Press, 1992.

Miller, Sarah D'Esti. "*Miss Saigon* Star Savors the Honesty of Live Theater." *Press and Sun-Bulletin,* 13 October 2005, http://www.presconnects.com/entettainment/stories.

"*Miss Saigon* Soon in RP." *Manila Mail Bayanihan,* December 2000: B5.

"*Miss Saigon* Watch: Equity Regained." *Los Angeles Times,* 17 August 1990: B6.

Moon, Katherine H. S. *Sex Among Allies: Military Prostitution in U.S.-Korea Relations*. New York: Columbia University Press, 1997.

Moon, Krystyn R. *Yellowface: Creating the Chinese in American Popular Music and Performance, 1850s–1920s*. New Brunswick, N.J.: Rutgers University Press, 2005.

Moore, Bill. "Asian Balm." *Other Stages* (April 1983), n.p.

Moore, Pamela L., ed. *Building Bodies*. New Brunswick, N.J.: Rutgers University Press, 1997.

Morris, Gay, ed. *Moving Words: Re-writing Dance*. New York: Routledge, 1996.

Moy, James S. "David Henry Hwang's *M. Butterfly* and Philip Kan Gotunda's *Yankee Dawg You Die*: Repositioning Chinese American Marginality on the American Stage." *Theatre Journal* 42, no. 1 (1990): 48–56.

——. *Marginal Sights: Staging the Chinese in America*. Iowa City: University of Iowa Press, 1993.

Muñoz, José Esteban. "Feeling Brown: Ethnicity and Affect in Ricardo Bracho's *The Sweetest Hangover (and Other STDs)*." *Theatre Journal: Latino Performance* 52, no. 1 (March 2000): 67–80.

Murphy, Jacqueline Shea. "Unrest and Uncle Tom: Bill T. Jones / Arnie Zane Dance Company's *Last Supper at Uncle Tom's Cabin / The Promised Land*." In *Bodies of the Text: Dance as Theory, Literature as Dance,* edited by Ellen W. Goellner and

Jacqueline Shea Murphy, 81–105. New Brunswick, N.J.: Rutgers University Press, 1994.

Murray, Karen. "Canadian Dream: *Saigon* Recoups in Just 161 Days." *Variety,* 18 October 1993: 61.

——. "Toronto Picketers Target *Miss Saigon.*" *Variety,* 7 June 1993: 47.

My America, or Honk If You Love Buddha. Directed by Renee Tajima-Pena. National Asian American Telecommunications Association (NAATA) in association with the Independent Television Service (ITVS), 1997.

Narita, Jude. *Walk The Mountain.* Highways Performance Space, Santa Monica, California. January 2002.

"Narrow Broadway." Editorial. *Christian Science Monitor,* 13 August 1990: 20.

Ness, Sally Ann. *Body, Movement, and Culture: Kinesthetic and Visual Symbolism in a Philippine Community.* Philadelphia: University of Pennsylvania Press, 1992.

——. "Dancing in the Field: Notes from Memory." In *Corporealities: Dancing Knowledge, Culture and Power,* edited by Susan Leigh Foster, 129–55. New York: Routledge, 1996.

"News Briefs." *A. Magazine* (June/July 2001): 14.

Newton, Rosemary. "Choreographer of the Month: Saeko Ichinohe." *Attitude: The Dancer's Monthly* 2, no. 3 (August 1983): 10.

Ngô, Fiona I.B. "The Anxiety Over Borders." In *Embodying Asian American Sexualities,* edited by Gina Masequesmay and Sean Metzger, 89–104. Lanham, Md.: Lexington Books, 2009.

Nguyen, Hung, et al., *Laughter From the Children of War.* Unpublished manuscript, 1997.

Nietzsche, Friedrich. *On the Genealogy of Morals and Ecce Homo.* 1967. Translated by Walter Kauffman and R. J. Hollingdale. New York: Vintage Books, 1989.

Nightingale, Benedict. "Where the Season Shines Brightest; *Miss Saigon* Is Hottest London Ticket." *New York Times,* 8 October 1989: sec. 5: 15+.

Novack, Cynthia J. *Sharing the Dance: Contact Improvisation and American Culture.* Madison: University of Wisconsin Press, 1990.

O'Keefe, Margaret. "Asian American Dance Theatre." *Attitude: The Dancer's Monthly* 2, no. 1 (June 1983): 10.

Okely, Judith, and Helen Callaway, eds. *Anthropology and Autobiography.* New York: Routledge, 1992.

Omi, Michael, and Howard Winant. *Racial Formation in the United States: From the 1960s to the 1990s.* 2nd ed. New York: Routledge, 1994.

Pai, Fei-lan. "Singing Across the Pacific: *Miss Saigon* and *Making Tracks.*" Master's thesis, University of Illinois–Urbana-Champaign, 2007.

Pang, Cecilia J. "Theater Departments Can Help Combat the Dearth of Asian Americans in the Entertainment Industry." Editorial. *Chronicle of Higher Education* (17 April 1991): B1+.

Pao, Angela. "Changing Faces: Recasting National Identity in All-Asian(-)American Dramas." *Theatre Journal* 53, no. 3 (2001): 389–409.

———. "The Eyes of the Storm: Gender, Genre and Cross-Casting in *Miss Saigon*." *Text and Performance Quarterly* 12 (January 1992): 21–39.

Peacock, James. *Rites of Modernization: Symbols and Social Aspects of Indonesian Proletarian Drama*. Chicago: University of Chicago Press, 1968.

Pennsylvania Ballet. Advertisement. *Philadelphia Metro,* 16–18 November 2001: 15.

Phelan, Peggy. *Unmarked: The Politics of Performance*. New York: Routledge, 1993.

Piedrafite, Joe. "The Last Night of the World: *Miss Saigon* Lands in Amherst." *Daily Collegian,* 13 October 2005, http://www.dailycollegian.com/vnews/display.v?T ARGET

Pratt, Mary Louise. *Imperial Eyes: Travel Writing and Transculturation*. New York: Routledge, 1992.

Prendiville, Callie. "Miss Saigon." *Orange County Register*, 27 March 2007, http://www.ocregister.com/ocregister/life/education/cappies/article_1632646.php.

Puccini, Giacomo. *Madam Butterfly, Madama Butterfly: Opera Guide 26,* edited by Nicholas John. New York: Riverrun Press, 1984.

Quindlan, Anna. "Public and Private; Error, Stage Left." *New York Times,* 12 August 1990, sec. 4, p. 21.

Rahman, Sukanya. *Dancing in the Family.* Delhi, India: Harper Collins, 2001.

Rabinow, Paul, ed. *The Foucault Reader*. New York: Pantheon Books, 1984.

Rand, Erica. *Barbie's Queer Accessories*. Durham, N.C.: Duke University Press, 1995.

Reed-Danahay, Deborah E., ed. *Auto/Ethnography: Rewriting the Self and the Social*. New York: Berg, 1997.

Reinelt, Janelle G., and Joseph R. Roach, eds. *Critical Theory and Performance*. Ann Arbor: University of Michigan Press, 1992.

Remen, Kathryn. "The Theater of Punishment: David Henry Hwang's *M. Butterfly* and Michel Foucault's *Discipline and Punish*." *Modern Drama* 37, no. 3 (1994): 391–400.

Resnikova, Eva. "Eastern Standard." *National Review* (17 September 1990): 51–54.

———. "Good Times Off Broadway." *National Review* (12 August 1991): 56.

Retamar, Roberto Fernández. *Caliban and Other Essays*. Translated by Edward Baker. Minneapolis: University of Minnesota Press, 1989.

Rich, Frank. "Jonathan Pryce, *Miss Saigon* and Equity's Decision." *New York Times,* 10 August 1990: C1+.

Richards, David. "The *Saigon* Picture Is Worth 1,000 Words." *New York Times,* 21 April 1991, sec. 2, p. 5+.

Rony, Fatimah Tobing. *The Third Eye: Race, Cinema, and Ethnographic Spectacle.* Durham, N.C.: Duke University Press, 1996.

Rothstein, Mervyn. "Dispute Settled, *Miss Saigon* Is Broadway Bound." *New York Times,* 19 September 1990: C11.

——. "Equity Council Approves Accord on *Miss Saigon.*" *New York Times,* 18 September 1990: C14.

——. "Equity Panel Head Criticizes *Saigon* Producer." *New York Times,* 16 August 1990: C15+.

——. "Equity Plans to Meet on Thursday." *New York Times,* 11 August 1990: sec. 1: 16.

——. "Equity Proposes Panel on *Miss Saigon* Role." *New York Times,* 12 December 1990: C18.

——. "Equity Reverses *Saigon* Vote and Welcomes English Star." *New York Times,* 17 August 1990: A1+.

——. "Equity Will Reconsider *Miss Saigon* Decision." *New York Times,* 10 August 1990: C3.

——. "Filipino Actress Allowed in *Saigon.*" *New York Times,* 8 January 1991: C11.

——. "MacKintosh and Equity Plan Meeting." *New York Times,* 24 August 1990: C3.

——. "*Miss Saigon* Takes on Equity Again." *New York Times,* 5 December 1990: C18.

——. "Producer Cancels *Miss Saigon*; 140 Members Challenge Equity." *New York Times,* 9 August 1990: C15+.

——. "Producer Demands a Free Hand to Cast *Miss Saigon* Roles." *New York Times,* 22 August 1990: C11–12.

——. "Scores of Actors Flock to Tryouts for Ethnic Roles in *Miss Saigon.*" *New York Times,* 2 October 1990: C11.

——. "Union Bars White in Asian Role; Broadway May Lose *Miss Saigon.*" *New York Times,* 8 August 1990: A1+.

——. "*Will Rogers* and *Saigon* Top Tony Race." *New York Times,* 7 May 1991: C13+.

——. "The Musical Is Money to His Ears." *New York Times Magazine,* 9 December 1990: 48+.

Royston, Peter, and Sarah Schlesinger. "*Miss Saigon" Study Guide*, edited by Helen Sneed. New York: Music Theatre International, 2000.

Russel, John. "Race and Reflexivity: The Black Other in Contemporary Japanese Mass Culture." In *Rereading Cultural Anthropology,* edited by George Marcus, 296–318. Durham, N.C.: Duke University Press, 1992.

Russo, Mary. *The Female Grotesque: Risk, Excess, and Modernity.* New York: Routledge, 1994.

Rutledge, Paul James. *The Vietnamese Experience in America.* Bloomington: Indiana University Press, 1992.

Safire, William. "Essay: Some Enchanted *Saigon.*" *New York Times,* 2 October 1989: A19.

Said, Edward W. *Culture and Imperialism*. New York: Vintage Books, 1993.

———. *Orientalism*. New York: Vintage Books, 1979.

———. "Representing the Colonized: Anthropology's Interlocutors." *Critical Inquiry* 15, no. 2 (1989): 205–25.

"*Saigon* Producer Seeks Arbitration." *New York Times,* 14 December 1990: C4.

Saito, Leland T. *Race and Politics: Asian Americans, Latinos, and Whites in a Los Angeles Suburb*. Urbana: University of Illinois Press, 1998.

Sardar, Ziauddin. *Postmodernism and the Other: The New Imperialism of Western Culture*. Chicago: Pluto Press, 1998.

Savigliano, Marta E. *Angora Matta: Fatal Acts of North-South Translation*. Middletown, Conn.: Wesleyan University Press, 2003.

———. "Nocturnal Ethnographies: Following Cortázar in the Milongas of Buenos Aires." *Etnorfoor* 10 (1997): 28–52.

———. "Tango and Its Postmodern Uses of Passion." In *Cruising the Performative,* edited by Sue-Ellen Case, Philip Brett, and Susan Leigh Foster, 130–48. Bloomington: University of Indiana Press, 1995.

———. *Tango and the Political Economy of Passion*. Boulder, Colo.: Westview Press, 1995.

Schafer, John C. "Trịnh Công Sơn Phenomenon." *Journal of Asian Studies* 66, no. 3 (August 2007): 597–643.

Schlesinger, Arthur Jr. "Same Difference." *American Theatre* (April 1993): 64.

Schlundt, Christina. *Daniel Nagrin: A Chronicle of His Professional Career*. Berkeley: University of California Press, 1997.

Schutzman, Mady, and Jan Cohen-Cruz, eds. *Playing Boal: Theatre, Therapy, Activism*. New York: Routledge, 1994.

Scott, Anna Beatrice. "Spectacle and Dancing Bodies that Matter: Or, If It Don't Fit, Don't Force It." In *Meaning in Motion: New Cultural Studies of Dance*, 259–68. Durham, N.C.: Duke University Press, 1997.

Seligman, Daniel. "A Boo for *Miss Saigon*." *Fortune* (8 October 1990): 187–88.

Shay, Anthony. *Choreophobia: Solo Improvised Dance in the Iranian World*. Costa Mesa, Calif.: Mazda Publishers, 1999.

Shelton, Suzanne. *Divine Dancer: A Biography of Ruth St. Denis*. Garden City, N.Y.: Doubleday, 1981.

Shimakawa, Karen. "'I'll be here . . . right where you left me': Mimetic Abjection/ Mimetic Mimicry." In *National Abjection: The Asian American Body Onstage*, 99–128. Durham, N.C.: Duke University Press, 2002.

———. "'Who's to Say?' Or, Making Space for Gender and Ethnicity in *M. Butterfly*." *Theatre Journal* 45, no. 3 (1993): 349–62.

———. "'Whose history is this anyway?' Changing Geographies in Ping Chong's *East-West Quartet*." In *National Abjection: The Asian American Body on Stage*, 129–39. Durham, N.C.: Duke University Press, 2002.

Shimizu, Celine Parreñas. "The Bind of Representation: Performing and Consuming Hypersexuality in *Miss Saigon*." *Theatre Journal* 57, no. 2 (May 2005): 247–65.

Siegel, Marcia B. *The Tail of the Dragon: New Dance, 1976–1982*. Durham, N.C.: Duke University Press, 1991.

Simon, John. "Leaden Butterfly." Review of *Miss Saigon*, music by Claude-Michel Schönberg, book by Alain Boublil and Claude-Michel Schönberg, lyrics by Alain Boublil and Richard Maltby Jr. Broadway Theatre, New York. *New York Magazine*, 22 April 1991: 76+.

Smith, Chris. "Mr. Saigon: Jonathan Pryce Takes on the Part and the Controversy of a Lifetime in Broadway's Most Expensive Musical." *New York Magazine*, 11 March 1991: 47+.

Smith, Dinitria. "Face Values: The Sexual and Racial Obsessions of Playwright David Henry Hwang." *New York Magazine*, 11 January 1993: 40+.

Song, John Huey, and John Dombrink. "'Good Guys' and Bad Guys: Media, Asians, and the Framing of a Criminal Event." *Amerasia* 22, no. 3 (1996): 25–45.

Sontag, Susan, ed. *A Barthes Reader*. New York: Hill and Wang, 1982.

Spelman, Elizabeth V. *Inessential Woman: Problems of Exclusion in Feminist Thought*. Boston: Beacon Press, 1988.

Spivak, Gayatri Chakravorty. "Can the Subaltern Speak?" In *Marxism and the Interpretation of Culture*, edited by Cary Nelson and Lawrence Grossberg, 271–313. Urbana: University of Illinois Press, 1988.

——. *In Other Worlds: Essays in Cultural Politics*. New York: Routledge, 1988.

Srinivasan, Priya. "The Bodies Beneath the Smoke or What's Behind the Cigarette Poster: Unearthing Kinesthetic Connections in American Dance History." In *Discourses in Dance* 4, no. 1 (2007): 7–48.

——. "The Nautch Women Dancers of the 1880s: Corporeality, U.S. Orientalism and Anti-immigration Laws." *Women and Performance* 19, no. 1 (March 2009): 3–22.

——. "South Asian Cultural Performances: Inscribing Identities on the Diasporic Bodies." Paper presented at Congress on Research and Dance. Pomona, California, 4 December 1999.

Stam, Robert, and Ella Shohat. *Unthinking Eurocentrism: Multiculturalism and the Media*. London: Routledge, 1994.

Stoler, Ann Laura. *Race and the Education of Desire: Foucault's "History of Sexuality" and the Colonial Order of Things*. Durham, N.C.: Duke University Press, 1995.

Stone, Robert. "*Miss Saigon* Flirts with Art and Reality." *New York Times*, 7 April 1991, sec. 2, p. 1+.

Straub, Kristina. *Sexual Suspects: Eighteenth-Century Players and Sexual Ideology*. Princeton, N.J.: Princeton University Press, 1992.

Strauss, Sarah. *Positioning Yoga: Balancing Acts Across Culture*. Oxford: Berg Publishers, 2005.

Studlar, Gaylyn. "Out-Salomeing Salome: Dance, the New Woman, and Fan Magazine Orientalism." In *Visions of the East: Orientalism in Film,* edited by Matthew Bernstein and Gaylyn Studlar, 99–129. New Brunswick, N.J.: Rutgers University Press, 1997.

Suh, Mary. "The Many Sins of *Miss Saigon*." *Ms.* (December 1990): 63.

Sun, Shirley. "For Asians Denied Asian Roles, 'Artistic Freedom' Is No Comfort." . *New York Times,* 26 August 26 1990: H7+.

Takaki, Ronald. *Strangers from a Different Shore: A History of Asian Americans.* New York: Penguin Books, 1990.

"Talks on *Miss Saigon* Are Continuing." *New York Times,* 23 August 1990: C24.

Taussig, Michael. *Mimesis and Alterity: A Particular History of the Senses.* New York: Routledge, 1993.

Taylor, Diana, and Juan Villegas, eds. *Negotiating Performance: Gender, Sexuality, and Theatricality in Latin/o America.* Durham, N.C.: Duke University Press, 1994.

Terry, Walter. *Miss Ruth: The More Living Life of Ruth St. Denis.* New York: Dodd, Mead, 1969.

"This Is Equity?" Editorial. *Washington Post,* 15 August 1990: A20.

Thomas, Helen., ed. *Dance in the City.* New York: St. Martin's Press, 1997.

Thomson, Rosemarie Garland, ed. *Freakery: Cultural Spectacles of the Extraordinary Body.* New York: New York University Press, 1996.

Thornton, Sarah. *Club Cultures: Music, Media, and Subcultural Capital.* Hanover, N.H.: University Press of New England, 1996.

Tran, Barbara, Monique T. D. Truong, and Luu Truong Khoi, eds. *Watermark: Vietnamese American Poetry and Prose.* New York: Asian American Writers Workshop, 1998.

Trinh, T. Minh-ha. *When the Moon Waxes Red: Representation, Gender and Cultural Politics.* New York: Routledge, 1991.

———. *Woman, Native, Other: Writing Postcoloniality and Feminism.* Bloomington: Indiana University Press, 1989.

Tsai, Shih-shan Henry. *The Chinese Experience in America.* Bloomington: Indiana University Press, 1986.

Tsing, Anna Lowenhaupt. *In the Realm of the Diamond Queen: Marginality in an Out-of-the-Way-Place.* Princeton, N.J.: Princeton University Press, 1993.

"Two Stage Triumphs." Editorial. *New York Times,* 18 August 1990, sec. 1, p. 24.

Tucker, Robert C., ed. *The Marx-Engels Reader.* 2nd ed. New York: W. W. Norton, 1972.

Uno, Roberta. *Unbroken Thread: An Anthology of Plays by Asian American Women.* Amherst: University of Massachusetts Press, 1993.

Van Meter, Jonathan. "Broadway Baby." *Vogue* (June 1991): 178+.

Visweswaran, Kamala. *Fictions of Feminist Ethnography*. Minneapolis: University of Minnesota Press, 1994.

Walter, Kathy. "Spotlight Students Become Pioneers in Musical Theater." *Your North Hills*, 18 April 2007, www.yournorthhills.com/node/1745.

West, Cornel. *Race Matters*. New York: Vintage Books, 1994.

West, Philip, Steven I. Levine, and Jackie Hiltz, eds. *America's Wars in Asia: A Cultural Approach to History and Memory*. New York: M. E. Sharpe, 1998.

White, Hayden. *The Content of the Form: Narrative Discourse and Historical Representation*. Baltimore, Md.: Johns Hopkins University Press, 1987.

Whitney, Craig R. "America's Vietnam Trauma Is the Stuff of British Musical." *New York Times*, 23 September 1989: sec. 1: 12.

Wiegman, Robyn. *American Anatomies: Theorizing Race and Gender*. Durham, N.C.: Duke University Press, 1994.

Will, George. "A Degradation of American Liberalism." *Los Angeles Times*, 13 August 1990: B7

———. "The Trendy Racism of Actors' Equity." *Washington Post*, 12 August 1990: C7.

Willet, John, ed. and trans. *Brecht on Theatre: The Development of an Aesthetic*. 1957. New York: Hill and Wang, 1964.

Winfield, Paul. "Equity Was Right the First Time." Editorial. *New York Times*, 18 August 1990, sec. 1, p. 25.

Witchel, Alex. "Actors' Equity Attacks Casting of *Miss Saigon*." *New York Times*, 26 July 1990: C18.

———. "British Star Talks of Racial Harmony and Disillusionment with Equity." *New York Times*, 11 August 1990, sec. 1, p. 15+.

———. "The Iron Butterfly within *Miss Saigon*." *New York Times*, 17 March 1991, sec. 2, p. 5+.

———. "On Stage, and Off." *New York Times*, 27 March 1992: C2.

———. "Union Weighs *Miss Saigon* Casting." *New York Times*, 25 July 1990: C12.

Wong, Deborah. *Speak It Louder: Asian Americans Making Music*. New York: Routledge, 2004.

Wong, Yutian. "Discussion." In *Maps of City and Body*, edited by Denise Uyehara, 153–63. New York: Kaya Press, 2003.

———. "Towards a New Asian American Dance Theory." *Discourses in Dance* 1, no. 1 (2002): 69–89.

Woo, Deborah. "The Gap Between Striving and Achieving: The Case of Asian American Women." In *Making Waves: An Anthology of Writings by and about Asian American Women*, edited by Asian Women United of California, 185–94. Boston: Beacon Press, 1989.

Woo, Michelle. "What's It Like to Work with Fingers and Toes?" *Nguoi Viet 2*

Online, 12 February 2004; http://nguoi-viet.com/absolutenm/anmviewer.asp?a =705&z=43.

Wray, Matt, and Annalee Newitz, eds. *White Trash: Race and Class in America*. New York: Routledge, 1997.

Xing, Jun. *Asian America through the Lens: History, Representations, and Identity*. Walnut Creek, Calif.: Altamira Press, 1998.

Yamamoto, Traise. *Masking Selves, Making Subjects: Japanese American Women, Identity, and the Body*. Berkeley: University of California Press, 1999.

Yoshihara, Mari. *Embracing the East: White Women and American Orientalism*. New York: Oxford University Press, 2003.

Yoshikawa, Yoko. "The Heat is on *Miss Saigon* Coalition: Organizing Across Race and Sexuality." In *The State of Asian America: Activism and Resistance in the 1990s*, edited by Karin Aguilar-San Juan, 275–94. Boston: South End Press, 1994.

Yung, Judy. *Unbound Feet: A Social History of Chinese Women in San Francisco*. Berkeley: University of California Press, 1995.

INDEX

ABOUT THE AUTHOR

Yutian Wong is Assistant Professor of Dance at the San Francisco State University. Her publications include the essay "Discussion," in *Maps of City and Body* by Denise Uyehara (Kaya Press, 2003), and the essay "Towards a New Asian American Dance Theory: Locating the Dancing Asian American Body," in *Discourse in Dance* 1.1 (2002). She was a member of Club O' Noodles, a Los Angeles–based Vietnamese American art collective, from 1996 to 2000.